2 MINUTES TO
Sleep

2 MINUTES TO
Sleep

Everyday Self-Care
for a Better Night's Rest

Corinne Sweet

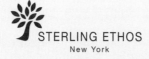

STERLING ETHOS
New York

Forever grateful to my late father, Leslie Sweet, for tucking me in at night to quell my fears and help me sleep with bedtime tales of his amazing seafaring days.

STERLING
New York

An Imprint of Sterling Publishing Co., Inc.
122 Fifth Avenue
New York, NY 10011

ISBN 978-1-4549-4298-6

Distributed in Canada by Sterling Publishing Co., Inc.
c/o Canadian Manda Group, 664 Annette Street, Toronto, Ontario M6S 2C8, Canada

For information about custom editions, special sales, and premium and corporate purchases, please contact Sterling Special Sales at 800-805-5489 or specialsales@sterlingpublishing.com.

Manufactured in Slovakia

10 9 8 7 6 5 4 3 2 1

sterlingpublishing.com

Cover design by Andrew Smith
Cover illustration by Lylean Lee
Interior design by Ginny Zeal
Interior illustration by Andrew Pinder

MIX
From responsible sources
FSC
www.fsc.org
FSC® C022120

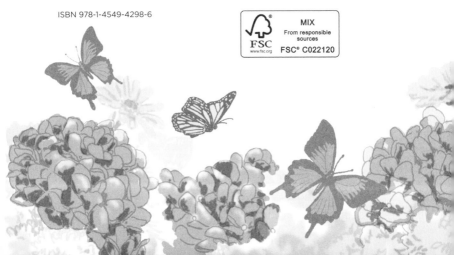

Contents

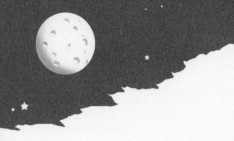

CHAPTER ONE

An Introduction to Sleep

How well did you sleep last night?
How did you feel on waking this morning?
Are you worried about getting enough sleep?
Did you spend ages trying to drop off?
Did you nap during the day and then wake up
in the middle of the night?
Was your sleep interrupted by young children or pets?
Are you finding that you are needing less
sleep at night and more naps during the day?
Did you have a nightcap to get to sleep?
Do you take sleeping pills?
Do you feel constantly tired?
Can you remember your dreams?

Sleep Deprivation

Sleep is a major preoccupation for many of us. We need sleep to regenerate and recover from our increasingly busy days, yet we are generally more sleep-deprived than ever before. The World Health Organization (WHO) has declared a sleep epidemic in industrialized nations. Most people in industrialized countries are getting less than the recommended eight to nine hours a night recommended by WHO for good physical and mental health. People living in Japan, Singapore, and Brazil are the most sleep-deprived, sleeping for an average of five to six hours a night, while those living in the Netherlands and New Zealand are getting the most sleep—around eight to ten hours a night.

Insomnia

Many people suffer from bouts of insomnia (not being able to sleep), which can be linked to physical and/or psychological issues borne of their lifestyle. Insomnia is dangerous to ourselves and others, as we often fail to function well the next day and complete daily tasks: driving cars, managing children, using machinery, even just crossing the road. We are awake for two-thirds of our lives, but we also need sleep time to recuperate and reboot our overloaded brains and bodies (see page 49).

What Is Sleep For?

William Shakespeare's famous quote from Macbeth, *"Sleep that knits up the ravell'd sleave of care,"* reflects the essential healing nature of sleep. Quality sleep is the *"chief nourisher in life's feast."* We all need sleep to restore and repair our bodies and brains after being awake and active for an average of sixteen to eighteen hours every day.

When we are awake, our brain waves are at their highest activity levels and our muscles are largely active. During sleep, our bodies restore themselves by releasing growth hormones, which repair cells. Our brains reboot as our brain waves slow down, and a huge amount of complex neurophysiological and hormonal changes occur. We also store our memories and dream every night, which is how our brains sift through and make sense of our waking hour experiences.

Sleep Cycle

There are four main stages of a sleep cycle:

Stage 1: NREM (Non-Rapid Eye Movement Sleep). This is the lightest stage of sleep and mainly a transition from being awake to falling asleep. Each stage lasts for five to ten minutes, and if woken, you may not think you've been asleep yet.

Stage 2: NREM. This accounts for about 40 to 60 percent of our sleep time and allows our brains to consolidate memories and process experiences. Each stage lasts for around twenty minutes as our body temperature drops, and our breathing and heartrate become more more regular.

Stage 3: NREM. We spend around 5 to 15 percent of our sleep time in this deep sleep phase. Our muscles relax and our blood pressure and breathing rates drop. We are less responsive to the environment, and sleepwalking and bed-wetting can happen.

Stage 4: REM (Rapid Eye Movement Sleep). Our brains become more active and our eyes move rapidly. We spend about 20 percent of our sleep time in this stage. Our muscles are relaxed, so if we wake up, we feel we can't move.

During the night we go through four or five sleep cycles. Sleep begins in stage one, progresses to two and three, and might repeat stages two and three before entering REM, stage four. After REM, the body and brain returns to stage two, then three, and so on.

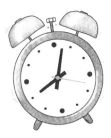

Why Are we Losing Sleep?

We are largely losing sleep due to the pressure of life and our 24/7 lifestyles. News is generated and available around the clock, which disturbs our emotional equilibrium. We are traveling more by airplane, driving long distances, and commuting to work, so we might have jet lag or the need to recover from a journey. Plus, we are working longer hours with more overtime and weekend work. Our nonstop economy has high expectations and constant needs to be met.

Sleep Needs

Generally, women need about 20 minutes more sleep per night than men due to multitasking (brain recovery time), pregnancy, and menopause (hormone changes). Women usually sleep slightly more than men on average, but they also experience more sleep problems. However, mothers get an average of fifteen minutes less sleep a night than fathers, and parents get around thirty-four hours less sleep a year than non-parents due to interrupted nights (See Sleep and Children on pages 138–147). Interestingly, women report that they wake up in a worse mood than men during the week (except in Columbia, Portugal, and the Ukraine).

SLEEP REVIEW

Take a piece of paper and pen and jot down everything you can about your sleep patterns. Knowing more about yourself and what helps you sleep is a good place to start if you want to improve your sleep habits or sleep hygiene. Ask yourself: How many hours do you sleep a night on average? How do you get off to sleep? Do you remember your dreams? Do you find it hard or easy to wake up? Do you prefer sleeping alone or with someone? Are there pets in your bedroom? Do you look at screens in bed? What interferes with your sleep? Do you wake up during the night, and if so, how many times? What do you eat or drink before bed? Take a minute to review your notes and consider what changes might be needed to achieve better sleep.

Writing exercise

How Does Sleep Loss Affect You?

If you don't get enough sleep at night, there are some key psychological side effects, such as:

- *Increased stress*
- *Forgetfulness*
- *Low mood*
- *Tiredness*
- *Lack of motivation*

Do you notice anything else, particular to you, such as being snappy, grumpy, or eating more carbohydrates?

There are also some negative physiological side effects, such as:

- *Respiratory problems*
- *Heart disease*
- *Diabetes*
- *Obesity*

As these side effects of sleep deprivation can affect our health and well-being, it is hugely important that we prioitize sleep and allow our bodies and minds adequate downtime.

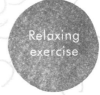

CLOUD SPOTTING

Try this anytime you are feeling stressed or can't sleep. If it is daytime, go and find a window, or look up into the sky. Can you see any clouds? Notice their color, shape, height, and spread. Are they dark gray, light gray, white, puffy, layered? If it is nighttime, can you see any clouds in the sky—are they moonlit? What color are they? What are the shapes?

Lifestyle Shifts

With one in two marriages breaking down, children might well end up being the responsibility of one parent. Being on duty at work and at home can really affect your sleep after a busy day. Plus, relationship breakdowns generally cause heartache and sleepless nights for everyone concerned.

Noise has increased with growing population density and traffic, especially in inner cities. Light pollution from streets, stores, and vehicles can interrupt our sleeping patterns. Plus, we are glued to screens and devices day and night, which affects our brain waves and keep us awake and wired when we want and need to sleep. We are also eating and drinking late and consuming more alcohol and drugs, which can affect our sleep.

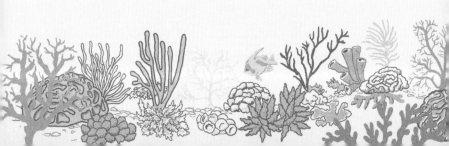

WALL STRETCH

Relaxing exercise

Take a break from what you are currently doing and find a clear space on a wall without any shelving, pictures, or light switches. Stretch upward toward the ceiling with your arms above your head, then turn to have your back to the wall. Stand with your body pressed against the wall—your buttocks, shoulders, and head touching. Your hands can touch the wall either side or hang by your sides. Your feet should be slightly away from the wall, hip-width apart. Push your lower back gently into the wall while keeping your head in contact with the wall, then relax. Push your lower back in again and repeat three more times.

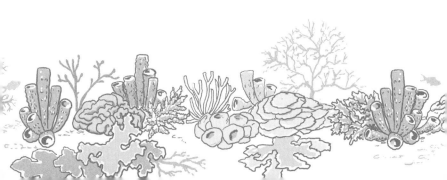

HEAD REST

Energizing exercise

If you are feeling groggy during the day, take a moment to rest your head. Try this sitting at a desk or table. Cup your hands together in front of you, as if you are catching water. Put your hands over your face, with your fingertips resting on your eyebrows, and the heel of your hands cupped under your chin. Your thumbs should be spread out to rest just under your ears. Put your elbows on the table or desk. Let your face rest gently in your hands for a couple of minutes. Notice how dark and relaxing it is. Close your eyes. Breathe in deeply and let your head rest on your own hands this way while you continue to breathe. Empty your mind as much as you can, focusing on the experience of resting your head on your hands. After a couple of minutes take your hands away, straighten up, and just sit for a few seconds.

HEAD ROLL

Relaxing exercise

Stand with your feet hip-width apart and your arms loose by your sides. Close your eyes and let your head drop forward gently, tucking your chin into your throat. Slowly roll your head to the left, then roll it back with your face tilted up to the ceiling. Repeat on the right side. Do this six times, breathing in and out slowly and calmly as you do. Notice any areas of tension or stiffness.

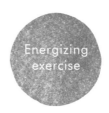

Energizing exercise

GOLDFISH STRETCH

This stretch is great if you are feeling tired or tense. Step away from your desk or stop what you are doing. Find a private space, such as your bedroom or the restroom, if you are at work. Sit or stand comfortably. Open your mouth wide and then purse your lips like a goldfish. Feel the stretch down the back of your neck as you do this. Open and close your mouth slowly six times, pausing in between. You may find yourself yawning as you relax—let the yawn happen. At the end, roll your head once to the left, once to the right, once backward, once forward. Then go back to what you were doing feeling energized and ready to continue the day.

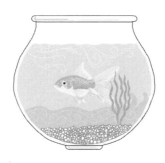

Sleep Moves

During sleep it is quite normal to wake intermittently, shift position, and move around. However, some people experience parasomnia behaviors, such as sleepwalking, sleep talking, night terrors, and bed-wetting. These can be a sign of emotional disturbance or physical discomfort, a result of age, or in some cases, down to genetics. These behaviors can disturb our sleep (and certainly disturb those around and next to us). Some of us will also experience loud snoring or sleep apnea, which can make sleeping very difficult for partners or children who are sleeping in the same room.

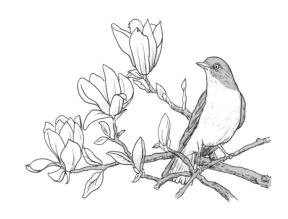

Relaxing exercise

SOUND AWARE

Sit back, stand, or walk around where you are. What can you hear? Really listen. Can you hear far away sounds? Immediate sounds? A dog barking? Traffic? Machinery? Water? A buzzing fly? Birdsong? Music? Notice the sounds. Are there any in your head, like tinnitus? Notice how far away things sound, or how near. Are they loud? Quiet? How do you feel when you really hear them? Take a deep breath and blow it out slowly once you are finished with noticing the sounds in your environment.

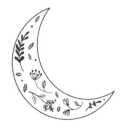

Sleep and Self-Care

Getting a good night's sleep is all about looking after yourself and your own well-being. Many of us get into bad habits around sleep, such as eating late, falling asleep in front of the television, or having an alcoholic nightcap to help us get to sleep. All of these things actually impair sleep rather than encourage a healthy dose of it. Deciding to look after yourself—and adopting a regular self-care regime—can really improve your sleep. It means you will gain knowledge about what suits you best, as an individual, and be able to give yourself what you need to achieve restful sleep.

Establish Self-Care Habits

Maximizing your self-care by allowing yourself time for two-minute breaks throughout your waking hours will really help to improve your sleep at night. It's not about napping constantly but rather about learning to do exercises (both for your mind and body) that will enhance your sleep.

By integrating self-care exercises into your daily life to boost your sleep, you can become more aware of yourself, of how you feel, and what you need. You need to know yourself well enough to stop and give yourself a boost whenever you are struggling. This is the essence of self-care: noticing when you are tense, overburdened, exhausted, worn out, wired, fed-up, or self-sabotaging, and learning to take a couple of minutes to relax, refocus, and do something positive for yourself. By changing your mood, you can take steps to change your situation.

Give Yourself Permission

Self-care is not a last-minute add-on; it is absolutely essential and needs to be fully integrated as a practice into our daily lives. Self-care should be a habit—like drinking more water or brushing your teeth. In fact, adding little acts of self-care onto our daily routines is a very good way of learning to weave it into the fabric of each day—such as stretching while at your desk or lying on the floor doing pelvic exercises while on the phone to friends. You just have to give yourself permission to do it. It's not a waste of time; it's essential and life-enhancing.

TAKE A BREAK

Sit or lie comfortably for a couple of minutes on your bed, couch, or the floor. Close your eyes. Take a moment to imagine yourself in the most relaxed position or place that you can imagine. It might be at a lovely sandy beach, on a purple chaise longue, in a wonderful bed, or on fresh green grass in a meadow. Imagine your surroundings: the sound of the sea lapping on the beach, or the smell of perfume and soft music as you recline on your chaise longue. Or being snuggled under a silky duvet in your comfy bed, or hearing the birds tweeting as you lie, feeling the sun on your body, in fragrant long grass surrounded by wildflowers. Imagine your scene and yourself, serene, at the center, spread out, and relaxed. After a couple of minutes, open your eyes, and see how you feel. Are you more relaxed?

Visualization exercise

SWEETEN THE MOMENT

Relaxing exercise

This mindfulness exercise will help you to slow down, relax, focus, and be more aware. If you like chocolate, take a square and put it on your tongue. Instead of eating it quickly, just let it melt slowly. Take your time to taste all the flavors, to experience the sensation in your mouth. Enjoy as you swallow, noticing the texture as it dissolves. If it has different constituents, like raisins or nuts, butterscotch or honeycomb, notice the sweet and sour qualities, the textures of these parts. Chew if you need, but continue to savor the chocolate until it has melted away.

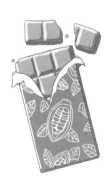

Two-Minute Sleep Booster

A two-minute break will refresh and reboot your
mind and body, and therefore your life. It will also help you
sleep better. Research shows that meditating daily (and several
times a day) will help to reduce muscle tension, headaches,
digestive conditions, and stress. You will increase your ability to
tackle new tasks as you oxygenate your blood and brain.
Endorphins, melatonin, growth hormones, oxytocin—the
feel-good chemicals released when we breathe deeply or
exercise—will help you to feel calmer and more in control.
Thus, a two-minute mental break can also help you face
the next challenges of the day.

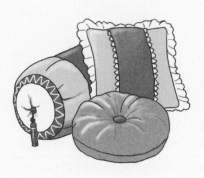

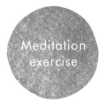

RISING AND FALLING

This can be done sitting or lying down (on an armchair, high-backed chair, beanbag, office chair, couch, back of the car, on the grass, on a beach, even in the restroom). Get yourself comfortable, turn off your cell phone, and set a timer for two minutes. Close your eyes and bring your focus to the middle of your forehead. As you breathe in think "rising," and as you breathe out think "falling." Keep your focus behind your forehead as you breathe in and out. Let go of any sounds you hear, and let your jaw loosen as you breathe. Drop your shoulders, feel your feet on the floor. Keep breathing, deepening the breath as you go. When the timer goes off, take a few moments before you open your eyes and set off again.

Mindful exercise

A MINDFUL COFFEE BREAK

Take a tea, coffee, or hot drink break. Decide to approach the whole exercise mindfully. Notice the water going into the kettle, and the sound of the kettle boiling. Or perhaps you have hot water from a machine at work. Put the tea bag or coffee in the cup, mug, or receptacle. When you pour over the hot water, notice the sound it makes. Then notice any changes in aroma, the steam, the smell. If you are making tea, notice how the tea comes out of the bag, its color. Then, however you take your tea or coffee, with milk or plain, with lemon or in a glass or mug, notice the color in the vessel before you drink it. Notice how it changes from a dense color to a lighter shade. When you take a sip, notice the taste on your tongue. Slow the whole process down for a couple of minutes to savor all your senses as you make your favorite hot drink.

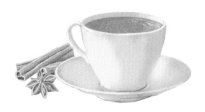

SPOT THE COLORFUL OBJECTS

Take a two-minute break and look around you at your office or your home, or out of a window. Can you spot ten objects that are blue? Notice them and say what they are to yourself. Then look for ten objects that are yellow. Again, say what they are to yourself. Take a deep breath in and out, then continue with your day. You can repeat this exercise with any color you like whenever you need a break.

Calming exercise

Mindful exercise

SLOW ORANGE PEEL

Take an orange and a sharp knife. Slice off a circle of peel at the naval and stem, then score the orange from the top to the bottom five times. Put your knife down and peel each section of peel from the top to the bottom— each panel of pith should come away easily. Enjoy your orange, savoring the taste and texture.

CHAPTER TWO

Sleep and Lifestyle

Sedentary and screen-based lifestyles are not conducive to getting a good night's sleep. When people rose early and ploughed the fields all day, or walked miles to work and did physically challenging labor, quality sleep was far easier to come by. Now we sit in cars, at desks, on couches, and increasingly rely on technology to run our lives. We use machines to do physically demanding jobs, and this is set to increase over time. Even gardening, chores, cooking, and car cleaning is beginning to be done by gadgets and robots, which are set to take over more and more physical tasks.

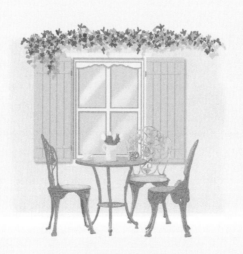

Lifestyle Factors

How well you sleep probably reflects how you live your life. Although most of us are craving a solid eight hours of bliss in a comfy bed, many of us end up having short, interrupted, and unsatisfactory nights. Always feeling tired and short of sleep has become a common preoccupation and topic of conversation. It's interesting to think that much of what we do today to ourselves might well be interfering with our ability to sleep and sleep enough. In other words, it can be a bit of a self-inflicted malaise. That's not to blame people, but to point out that we all may have slipped into unhealthy habits that are curbing our ability to have a good night's sleep. Luckily, there is plenty of information and research available to inform what we need to do to help ourselves.

CHILD'S POSE

Relaxing exercise

Take a moment away from your desk or stop what you are doing. Find a quiet corner or private space and get down on your knees. Sit back on your legs, then bend over and stretch your arms out along the floor, hands touching, with your head between your arms. Stretch, then rest. Repeat, remembering to breathe. Feel the stretch through your arms, back, and buttocks. Stretch again and rest. Sit up gently, roll your shoulders backward three times, and see how you feel.

QUICK LUNGE

Find a tabletop, countertop, or desk edge you can hold on to. Turn to face the surface with your feet hip-width apart and about two paces back from the edge of the surface. Lean toward the surface and hold on to it so your body bends from the waist with your arms out at full stretch. Tuck your bottom under, bend your legs, and move into a lunge position. Hold for a few moments. Slowly straighten your legs and return to standing. Make sure you tuck your behind under and bend your knees, lunging slowly, and without any pulls or pains. Repeat six times. Stand up and shake yourself out.

Energizing exercise

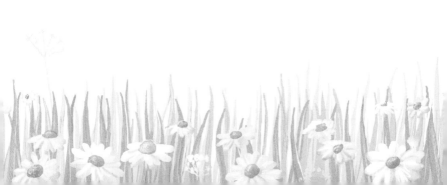

Physical and Physiological Factors Affecting Sleep

Many of us feel we simply don't get a good night's sleep. We are increasingly aware of the effects of work stress, screens, pressure, parenting, travel, and deadlines on our well-being, yet paradoxically our lifestyles often worsen our sleep quality. Although we are generally more health aware and many of us are living longer, we are still largely unaware of how our habits, hormones, and psychological states can affect our sleep.

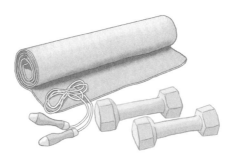

Work

Working long hours can keep us awake because it doesn't allow us time to wind down at the end of the day. Many of us will spend more time at work than in bed. Worrying about work can also keep us awake at night, especially if we take work to bed with us and our bedrooms are strewn with papers, files, gadgets, or laptops pinging and blinking away.

Lack of Exercise

Spending much of the day driving, commuting, and sitting at a desk without aerobic or cardiovascular exercise means we become more sluggish and less able to relax into sleep. However, exercising too near to bedtime can also keep us awake as we flood our bloodstreams with "feel-good" endorphins. It is recommended that vigorous exercise should take place before 9 p.m. to ensure we can relax into a good night's sleep. That said gentle exercise—such as stretches, yoga, and pilates—can help induce sleep,

Caffeine

Many of us are used to drinking large volumes of caffeinated tea and coffee throughout the day. Caffeine is also present in many other items, such as painkillers, fizzy drinks, and even ice cream. Caffeine is a powerful stimulant and if taken after 5 p.m. can affect sleep. Even decaffeinated coffee and tea are not entirely caffeine-free. Cutting down caffeine and not consuming caffeinated drinks or other products after 4.30 p.m. (and especially not during the hour before bed), should enhance your sleep.

Food

Long working hours and shift work often means that all too often the main meal of the day consists of rich, fatty food eaten late in the evening. This interferes with sleep as it overloads the digestive system and can be a hindrance to falling asleep. Plus, indigestion and gastric reflux can make us have to get up in the night for antacids because we are uncomfortable. Experts recommend that we avoid big meals after 8 p.m. Some foods, such as cereal and milk, or a warm milky drink can help us get to sleep but only in small quantities.

Alcohol

Alcohol interferes with sleep as it dehydrates our bodies. It is also a diuretic, so drinking alcohol in the evening will probably mean that you have to get up to go to the bathroom during the night. Alcohol might help you get to sleep, but it doesn't mean you'll get restful sleep. If you drink too much, your muscles relax, so you can end up snoring, which can be very disturbing to your partner (if you have one), children in your home, or even your neighbors.

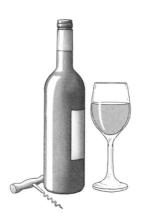

PICK AN ACTIVITY

Writing
exercise

Place a piece of plain paper on a table
horizontally. Fold the bottom left corner up to the
top edge and run your finger along the crease of
the paper. Tear or cut off the excess paper at the
right-hand margin, from top to bottom. You will have a square
piece of paper. Put the paper flat on the table, and fold in all four
corners in to meet at the center. You will have a square. Turn the
paper over. Fold in all four corners again to meet at the center.
Turn the paper over. Fold the paper in half, so you have two
squares each side with openings at the bottom. Keeping the paper
flat, slide your thumb and forefinger under the flap of paper, first
with your right hand. Then go to the other side of the square and
put your thumb and forefinger of your left hand under the flaps.

Put your thumb and fingers together in front of you. You will have
a paper object that opens one way and then the other when you
move your thumb and fingers back and forth. With a pen, write a
word outside of each square flap: the word can be something like
"swim," "dance," "nap," or "stretch."

Take your fingers out of the flaps, fold the paper back one stage, and write another word on each small triangle of paper inside, such as: "cup of tea," "rest," "smile," "breathe deeply" or "listen to a track."

Refold the paper as before, then put your thumb and fingers into the flaps. Move the paper backward and forward and then stop, without looking. See what your instructions are for a two-minute "pick a treat" break. Give yourself some fun. You can do this with a partner, child, or a friend, too. These are all nice things to do. Play this game with yourself when you feel you need a break.

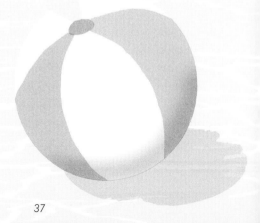

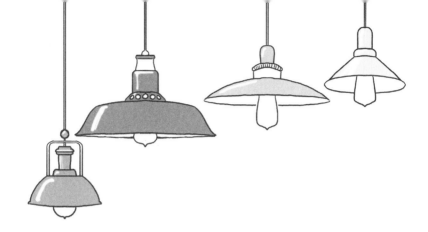

Environmental Factors Affecting Sleep

For many of us, our bedrooms double as an office, a game or computer room, a storeroom, or children's playground. They may be cluttered with clothes, laundry, pets, screens, and other daytime detritus. Most of the research on good sleep hygiene urges us to make our bedrooms a place of sanctuary for relaxation and peace. We need to eliminate clutter, reminders of our busy working lives, bright lights, environmental noise, and screens. Even the presence of pets and children need to be thought about carefully. The benefits of making adjustments to your bedroom—with sleep in mind—can improve your quality and quantity of rest no end.

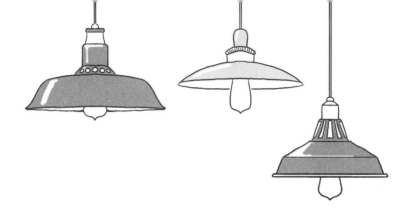

Room Temperature

If your bedroom is too hot, it can affect your ability to sleep. You will probably sweat, and this may cause some dehydration, meaning you will need a drink and subsequently may rewake needing go to the bathroom.

Light

When light enters the brain, it is a signal to wake up as adenosine, a neurochemical that helps rouse us for the day ahead, is released. If your drapes are flimsy, or your room is lit from outside, or from LEDs within, you may have an interrupted sleep. Try to make your room as dark as possible to enhance your sleep.

Noise

Even when you are asleep your brain still stays alert "listening" for predators and danger (it's how we survive). If you are in a noisy environment or have noise pollution from a loud neighbor with thumping music, clunking feet, rumbles from a road, vehicles, trains, a noisy refrigerator, or other disturbances, you will be on "red alert," unable to relax. This fills your bloodstream with cortisol and adrenalin, so you are in flight, fight, or freeze mode, rather than in a restful lets-go-to-sleep mode.

Mattress

Just like the story of the three bears, a mattress needs to be just right, neither too hard nor too soft. An overly firm mattress can interfere with sleep, especially if you have any back or joint problems; an over-soft mattress will not give you proper support, and may actually create or worsen any back problems.

Plus, the highly popular but expensive memory foam can be far too hot, interfering with your body's temperature by making you overheat. The best solution is probably a mix of springs, thin layers of memory foam, and other cotton-based materials to keep you cool and wick moisture away from you at night. Changing your mattress every eight years is recommended for health. You need to clean or even change your mattress regularly because the dust mites that inhabit your mattress cause rhinitis, asthma, and other symptoms, and sneezing and blocked sinuses can keep you awake at night.

Screens

Although watching TV in bed can feel like a luxury, a large, flickering screen can also interfere with sleep. Even though we now watch TV in all its forms on every kind of device—tablets, cell phones, laptops—the blue light from the screens interferes with our brain's ability to switch off and calm down. The blue light blocks the sleep-inducing hormone melatonin and keeps our brain waves buzzing. It therefore keeps us wide awake when we really want to sleep. The National Sleep Council suggests we block blue light and turn off screens for two to three hours before bedtime arrives.

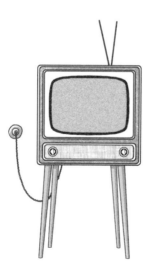

Pets on Beds

For some people, having their favorite cat, dog, pig, snake, or llama curled up on their bed is a recipe for a good, cuddly night. However, there are people for whom this is anathema. Pet hairs can cause allergies (and therefore sneezing); pet smells (especially dogs) can be disturbing; and pet movement can interrupt sleep. If you choose to have a pet with you, make sure your bed partner is happy about it. However, even if you love your pet's company, they may well be interfering with your (and your partner's) sleep, which you need to consider if you wish to sleep better.

Children in Bed

This can be a parental bone of contention. Many parents wish to have children in bed—called co-sleeping—even from babyhood, as it can mean the whole family can get a better night's sleep if one or both parents don't have to keep getting up. This is a very personal choice, however. There are guidelines on co-sleeping for babies as they need to sleep on their backs and at a relatively low temperature to stay safe. Being in a large, hot, adult bed may well be harmful to their health. You also need to be certain that your children are safe from being crushed or suffocated by adult bodies, bedding, or even pets. (See Sleep and Children, pages 138–147.)

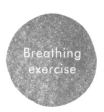

DIAPHRAGMATIC BREATHING EXERCISE

This exercise helps you relax and makes you more aware of your body during breathing. This can be good to do before bed, and makes a calming exercise first thing in the morning. Sit with your back against a wall and your legs crossed, or in a high-backed chair. Place one hand flat on your chest and the other on your solar plexus. Take a slow, deep breath through your nose, keeping your hand on your chest. Let your hand rise as you breath in and fall as you breath out. After three breaths, purse your lips and continue breathing, feeling the rise and fall in your belly. Notice the changes in your body as you breathe. Relax.

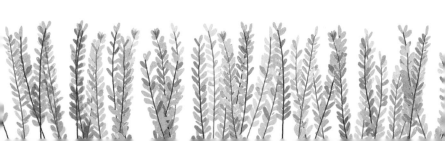

SELF-HUG STRETCH

Find a quiet space and stand with your feet hip-with apart. Stretch your arms out to the side, keeping your head upright. Bring your arms around your body with your right hand under your left armpit, and your left arm under your right armpit. Give yourself a hug. Squeeze and let go. Squeeze again. Take your arms out to the side again and repeat, left arm first. Do this three times.

Energizing exercise

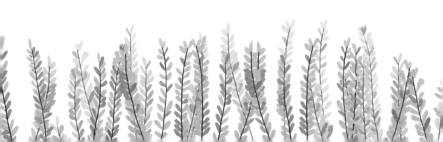

Acupressure
for Sleep

Acupressure works by stimulating the body's internal healing mechanisms and has been used in traditional Chinese medicine for over 3,000 years. Practicioners of Chinese medicine, including acupuncturists, accupressurists, shiatsu therapists, and reflexologists, can provide treatment to help with sleep disorders, but there are also exercises you can do at home by applying pressure to particular points on the body to aid relaxation and promote sleep.

1. Take your right index finger and feel the small hollow at the base of your left wrist, on the little finger side. Press your index finger gently into the hollow, and massage it for a minute or two.

2. Count four finger widths up from your ankle bone to the three yin intersection point just above the inside of your ankle. Apply deep pressure slightly behind your biggest leg bone, then massage in a circular motion for a few seconds.

3. Lie on your back and bend your knees. Take one foot in the opposite hand and feel the depression in the middle of the underside of the foot with your index finger—this is the bubbling spring point. Apply firm pressure and massage the point, using a circular up-and-down motion. Repeat with the other foot.

4. Turn your hands palms-up. Take your right hand and count three fingers down from your left wrist crease. With your right index finger, apply a steady pressure to the inner frontier gate between the two tendons. Then apply a circular up-and down motion for four to five seconds. Repeat on the other wrist.

5. Put both of your hands behind your head. Feel for the mastoid bone behind your ears and follow the groove to where your neck muscles attach to your skull with your fingers. Clasp your hands together and gently open your palms with your fingers interlocked in a cup-like shape. Use your thumbs to apply deep and firm pressure toward your skull, using circular and up-and-down movements. Do this for four or five seconds as you breathe deeply. This is known as the wind pool exercise and can reduce stress, calm your mind, and reduce any respiratory symptoms.

The Human Factor

Bedtime Habits

Some people can have the strangest of habits in bed, and it might be that your partner has bedtime habits that really drive you nuts—hogging the bedding, pummeling their pillows, you name it. A common annoying habit is checking cell phones and other devices constantly, even through the night. Another is snoring. Couples need to discuss these things as openly as possible to accommodate each other's particular bedtime proclivities (or at least, to tolerate and understand them). Lying awake stewing and resentful is never good for peaceful sleep.

Sleep Positions

When you are in a new relationship, it can be wonderful to be wrapped around each other in bed. Spooning is common (both people on their sides, facing in the same direction, one body pressed close to the other). However, over time, with familiarity and age, or when someone is ill or pregnant, people can begin to pull apart and sleep in their own styles. Some people like to lie spread-eagle across the bed or put their limbs outside the duvet, while others roll up in a fetal position. Sometimes keeping hold of the duvet becomes a tug of war. Then the depth of the duvet (whether it's a winter or summer one) becomes a bed-sharer's bone of contention: some like it hot, others don't. With all these things, talking and coming to some kind of working compromise is the answer.

Anxiety, Stress, and Insomnia

Nothing keeps us awake more than being anxious at night. Maybe you feel you can't turn your mind off. Or maybe you feel overloaded with too many worries and you can't fall asleep. Somehow, in the middle of the night, everything can seem very daunting. Often, when things are quiet and there are few distractions, we can end up feeling very alone and our worries seem enormous. Feeling anxious is very normal and let's face it; there seems to be a huge amount to worry about all the time in modern life. Insomnia can also be caused by a wide range of conditions, including physical illness, disability, hormonal changes, genetics, and even the magnetic pull of the moon.

MINDFUL DISHWASHING

Energizing exercise

Doing a household chore mindfully can offer a much needed mental break. If you have dishes to wash, pay attention to how you clean each object. Handle each item with attention, and wipe or scrub using a brush or sponge, enjoying the sensation of the hot water and the smell of the suds. Notice how things become clean. Enjoy the sense of getting something literally spick and span and then rinse. Notice the colors, the shiny surfaces, the bubbles. Then rinse off the soap and place the item on a drying rack. Continue with other dishwashing in a mindful manner.

STRETCH, FLOP, AND ROLL

Relaxing exercise

This is good to do either at bedtime or when getting up in the morning. Stand in an A frame shape with you legs hip-width apart. Raise both arms above your head in a gentle stretch, then let them flop down in front of you, as you bend over. Let your hands go down as far as they can go, even touch the floor. Stay there, with soft knees, for a few seconds. Roll gently up, vertebra by vertebra, until you are standing straight again. Pause and repeat three times. Relax.

CHAPTER THREE

Sleep and Screens

Fifty years ago, the only screens that people watched were usually either a fairly small television in the corner of the living room or a huge screen at the movies. Now, we are used to using and seeing screens from the minute we wake up until the end of the day (and even during the night). We are surrounded by screens all the time—they are everywhere and attached to our hands 24/7.

Screens have pervaded our lives, and we are all "screenagers" now with our cell phones, laptops, tablets, digital watches, timers, televisions, and smartphones. Children as young as babies and toddlers are screen-centerd, and there are plenty of silver surfers today too. As we move through each day, we move seamlessly from one screen to another, sometimes using several at once.

The End of the Day

Over the past twenty years, researchers have become both aware and concerned about how much our devotion to screens are affecting our brains. This is particularly important for us when we want to go to sleep, stay asleep, and wake up refreshed after a night of peaceful slumber. The average time it takes us to fall asleep is somewhere between ten and twenty minutes. It can take longer if we have drunk too much caffeine or alcohol, have eaten too much too late, are stressed, or have been using a screen right up until trying to go to sleep.

According to research most people go to bed between 10 and 11 p.m., with 20 percent going after midnight. If you have to be up at 6 or 7 a.m. and it takes a longer time to fall asleep, you are not going to get anywhere near a good eight hours of restful sleep.

 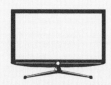

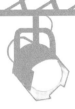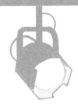

Blue Light

Going to bed is one thing; falling into a deep,
peaceful sleep is completely another. One of the biggest
culprits interfering with our sleep today is blue screen light. We
all have an internal biological clock, or a circadian rhythm,
which is what makes us wake up and governs our alertness
during the day. Although we are all unique, there is a fairly
common circadian pattern in human beings: light wakes us up
and the dark puts us to sleep.

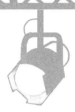
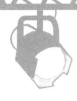

Sleep Drive

Our drive to sleep builds as the day continues toward its end and runs alongside the circadian rhythm, which dictates our body temperature as well as neurological and hormonal states. As we move toward evening, we get groggier and sleepier, which is called sleep inertia. This is nature's way of moving us toward wanting to go to sleep for the night.

The blue light on screens interferes with all of this. When we are looking at our screens right up until bedtime and during the night, our brain is woken up out of its groggy go-to-sleep state. Thus, blue light delays our internal body clock. It suppresses the release of melatonin, a hormone that helps us go to sleep, and increases adenosine, the hormone that wakes us up. When we finally hit the pillow, we can feel restless, irritable, wide awake, and unable to relax. Our brain waves are literally buzzing at high speed instead of slowing down.

Daytime Side Effects

We have specialized sensory cells in our retinas
that tell our brains whether it is night or day. Blue light from our
devices can cause confusing messages to reach our brains,
causing disrupted sleep patterns and sleep disorders. This
means we feel tired mid-morning and sleepy during the day
when we should, hopefully, be at our most alert and able to
work and function. There are serious issues around being safe
at the wheel of a car, dealing with children, or using machinery
at work, too.

MOLD A SHAPE

Try this if you are feeling anxious. Find some molding putty, polymer clay, or similar substance. Break off a chunk the size of a plum, or squish together several bits to make a ball. Soften it in your hands, rolling it in your palms. Then put the ball between your two palms and roll it around. Put the ball on a desk, tabletop, or keep it in your hands and see what you can make. A snowman or a cat? A vase or teapot? A snake or sausage? Let yourself play and enjoy shaping something using any props you have around, such as a pencil to make eye holes, or a paper clip for a hat. Sit back and admire your work.

Practical exercise

Sleep Hygiene

Some psychiatric research has shown sleep disorders caused by screen usage can be linked to the onset of depression and bipolar disorder. Experts call poor sleep habits bad sleep hygiene and encourage us all to think about the way we use our screens, including during the time leading up to bed and beyond.

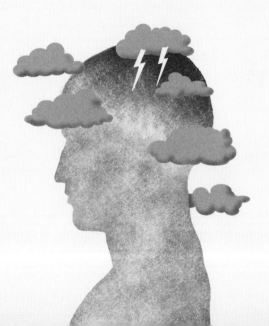

KNEELING STRETCH

Kneel on the floor in front of a couch, chair, table, or something you can hang on to. You might need a cushion under your knees. (You can also roll up a sweater, or use a coat for padding.) Check that your knees are directly under your hips and bend forward. Lengthening your spine, rest your forearms, palms-down, on the surface of the chair or couch seat, or along the table or stair. Let your head hang down slightly between your arms. Hold this stretch for a count of thirty. Then kneel upright and let your arms hang loosely by your side. Go back into the kneeling stretch, repeat, and then kneel upright. Do this a third time. Sit back on your heels and relax.

Stretching exercise

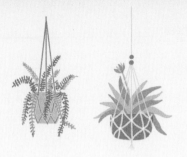
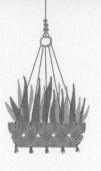
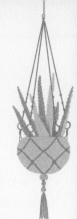

Health Issues

Health problems linked to the overuse of blue light from screens include breast and prostate cancer. This seems to be a result of the disruption of our circadian rhythm. Blue light also increases damage to our retinas and may bring on early macular degeneration and blindness. This is a condition that is usually associated with later life. Our eyes are very sensitive to light, obviously, as the visual photoreceptors, the rods (which provide night sight) and cones (which detect bright light and color), are needed to regulate our circadian responses.

In evolutionary psychology terms, our bodies have evolved over millennia to detect changes in light because it has been important for setting our body clocks. Being awake in the light meant we could hunt for food and fend off predators. The blue light we are all using is beginning to shift our body clocks and nobody really knows yet what the evolutionary outcome will be. However, the light can be quite addictive as we feel "high" rather than drowsy, forcing us to extend our days longer than our bodies and brains can really bear.

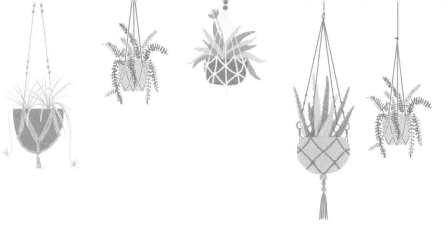

PREEN A HOUSEPLANT

Find a houseplant in your home or office. Concentrate on nurturing it for a moment: check for and remove any brown leaves. Feel the soil—does it need watering? Has the plant been fed recently? If not, add some plant feed to the water. Turn the plant in the light, so it has a different aspect. If you have a fine water spray, give it a spray. You could repeat this exercise with one or two plants in your house or office every time you need a break. A few minutes preening, pruning, plucking, and watering can give you a good mental break and improve your environment at the same time. Houseplants eat up carbon dioxide, so they are your healthy, inanimate indoor friends.

Practical
exercise

Self-Care and Screens

There are a few simple steps you can take to protect your and your family's eyes from blue screen light:

Specialist glasses: Protective glasses with a blue light filter are available from opticians or online.

Screen filters: There are screen filters available in all sizes to fit monitors or laptop screens.

Red light/blue light blockers: Most new smartphones, laptops, and other devices now come with an in-built blue light blocker or a red light filter. You can turn this on and change it to suit you by going to your settings. You can also download specialist blue light filtering apps (find one that is appropriate for your device and operating system).

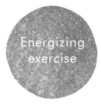

Energizing exercise

YAWN YOURSELF AWAKE

Find a private space and sit or stand comfortably. Open your mouth wide, really stretch it, and see if you can prompt a yawn. Wiggle your jaw to start the yawn and let it flow. When you yawn, you oxygenate your blood and relax muscle tension. Take a breath, open your mouth, widen, and wiggle your jaw and let the yawn come. Tears may roll down your cheeks. Enjoy the sensation. Stop and stretch and go back to where you were before, feeling newly refreshed.

Ten Tips for
Screen Sleep Hygiene

1. Take regular two-minute breaks away from your screens during the day to stretch, walk, relax, and rest your eyes.

2. If you work at a desk, get up and walk around every forty-five to sixty minutes. Stretch, talk to someone, make a drink, or pop outside.

3. Stop working on a screen for at least one or two hours before bed—screens and sleep don't mix.

4. Make sure your workstation is appropriate for your eyes in terms of height, screen distance, screen level in relation to your eyes, and that you have the right background lighting so you don't strain your eyes.

5. Ban gadgets from the bedroom or turn them off before you go to bed, including covering up any LED lights.

6. Don't bring your laptop or desktop into your bedroom.

7. Install a red light app on your computer and cell phone so that if you have to work late the color is warm and dimmed. This should help you sleep, even if you need to work late or use devices before bed (but it is not an excuse to work right up until bedtime).

8. Look up or away from your screen(s) regularly to let your eyes accommodate to the distant horizon (increased nearsightedness is at epidemic levels because we are looking down at close objects all the time). Looking at a distant horizon allows your lens to open and close and keeps your eyes healthy.

9. Ask any bed and bedroom sharers to turn off their screens and sounds so as not to disturb your sleep.

10. If you absolutely cannot avoid having screens or LED lights in your sleeping area, wear an eye mask to block out the light and use earplugs if you are very sensitive to noise.

Stretching exercise

GENTLE NECK STRETCH

Take a couple of minutes away from your desk or stop what you are doing and find a private place to sit comfortably. Take your right hand over the top of your head, to your left ear. Gently bring your right ear down toward your right shoulder. Hold this position for a five slow breaths in and out. Let go and straighten up. Bring your left hand over the top of your head, to your right ear. Bring your left ear down toward your left shoulder. Hold this position for five breaths in and out. Repeat, then sit upright and relax.

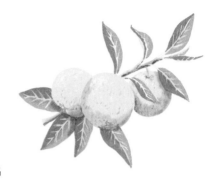

MINDFUL SNACKING

It's easy to nibble away at work on nuts, chocolate, cookies, and potato chips. Try to limit your eating to two-minute breaks. Wash your hands then get a raisin, a nut, some dried fruit, a piece of fresh fruit, like satsuma segments or bit of a banana, and eat one piece slowly. Try putting just one raisin, a segment of satsuma, or chunk of banana on your tongue. Close your mouth and let it warm up. Suck and eat it as slowly and awarely as you can. Savor the taste, the juice, the sensation as the fruit swells or dissolves, and simply relish a very slow mastication. Only swallow once you really have tasted all the flavors and experienced the changes in texture and shape.

Practical exercise

CHAPTER FOUR

Insomnia

"I can't sleep!" Many of us lie awake at night, staring at the ceiling, fidgeting, and shuffling in bed, trying to get comfortable to fall asleep. It can feel exhausting and isolating, trying to command sleep while feeling wide awake and restless in the dark. Research has found 40 to 50 percent of us suffer from sleep issues, and over a third experience insomnia. Plus, a huge 67 percent experience disrupted sleep, with 22 percent of us struggling to fall asleep each night. The most sleep-deprived countries are Singapore, Japan, and Brazil, and the best places to sleep are The Netherlands, New Zealand, and France. Americans are sleeping one hour less per night than in 1942, averaging 6.8 hours.

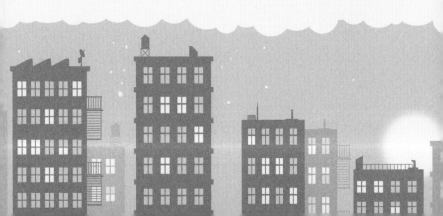

The Causes of Insomnia

In modern life, we have almost become accustomed to our sleep being interrupted and short (certainly less than eight hours), as a by-product of living fast, screen-centerd lives. Many of us long for a deep, nourishing sleep and to wake up refreshed and ready to go, yet we end up feeling tired all day instead. In fact, insomnia is usually the result of an underlying problem or set of problems. So if you are going to improve your sleep, you'll need to pinpoint exactly what is causing your sleepless nights. It may, of course, be a combination of things, but it's useful to understand your own lack-of-sleep cocktail so you can begin to do something about it.

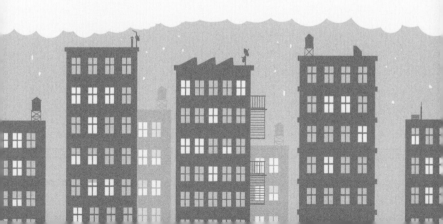

LONG BREATH EXERCISE

In private, get into a comfortable chair or sit on your bed. Take a long, deep breath in, then exhale fully, feeling what happens in your body as you do so. Breathe in and out three times in this way. Then take a breath in and slow your exhale down so that it is twice as long as your inhale. Do this twice. Stop and see how you feel.

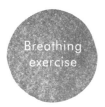

Breathing exercise

OUTSIDE MUNCH

Practical exercise

Try this at lunch time, after work, or simply when you need a break. Take a nice snack to eat and find a bench. Look at your surroundings and eat your snack slowly. Decide not to check your cell phone rather concentrate on the taste and texture of what you are eating. Notice the sky, the clouds, the trees, and how things taste in the open air. Taste every bit while you notice the air on your skin, the light, and any surroundings. When you have finished, sit for a few minutes just being.

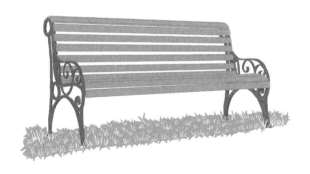

Types of Insomnia

Acute Insomnia
Usually a brief episode of not sleeping due to a life event such as stress, losing a job, divorce, an accident, bad news, or dealing with a difficult situation.

Chronic Insomnia
A persistent pattern of not sleeping lasting for three nights a week for longer than three months. This might be caused by trauma, especially PTSD (post traumatic stress disorder) or stress. It might include difficulty in falling asleep and staying asleep.

Comorbid Insomnia
Linked to psychiatric and psychological problems, such as anxiety and depression. It might also be linked with physical conditions such as painful arthritis, back pain, or a chronic medical condition.

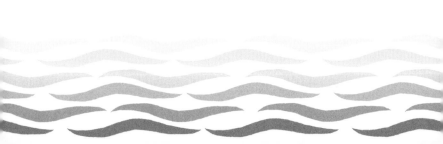

Onset Insomnia
Describes a difficulty with falling asleep at the beginning of the night. This may have many causes, but one might be the overuse of technology and screen-use with blue light (see Sleep and Screens, pages 52–67). It can also be linked to anxiety, stress, trauma, and painful childhood issues.

Maintenance Insomnia
Describes waking up in the night after having fallen asleep and then finding it difficult to get back to sleep. This can be due to stress and anxiety but also to hormonal changes (such as menopause), aging, alcohol, or drug use.

Postnatal Insomnia
Disrupted sleep patterns resulting from being woken by a crying baby for feeding or colic, or and postpartum hormonal changes. It might also be due to postnatal depression and exhaustion, tension, or stress of dealing with the demands of early parenthood.

SEATED FORWARD BEND

Try this at home or in a private place where there is floor space available. Sit down with your legs in front of you, pull in your tummy to lengthen your spine and press your hip bones into the floor. Bend your body forward over your legs, reaching your arms out in front of you. Tuck your chin into your chest and bend right over, holding your feet (if possible) with your hands, or resting them on your legs. Hold this pose for a couple of minutes, then relax. Afterward, lie on the floor and notice how your body is now feeling.

Relaxing exercise

ENJOY A SLOW TRACK

Relaxing exercise

Get comfortable on the couch, in bed, on the floor, or in a field. Put on a track of something slow, soothing, instrumental, or vocal. Stretch your body out with your back to the floor, and just listen. Enjoy the sounds and let the music fill your mind and body. Let the sound waves wash over you. Just enjoy the slowness, voices, instruments, and musical tones.

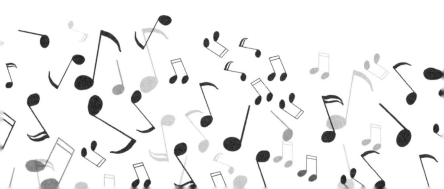

Seven Deadly Foes of a Good Night's Sleep

While some lucky people flop into bed and fall asleep the minute their heads touch the pillow, it's a different story for about 60 percent of us. We may approach the night with a sense of foreboding—exhausted but unable to sleep. We might even feel too tired and overwhelmed to begin to wind down and keep ourselves awake by binge-watching TV or scrolling on our cell phones and laptops. Or maybe we try and relax by gaming or drinking alcohol, only to find sleep escapes us until dawn. The first step to getting enough sleep is to understand what prevents it.

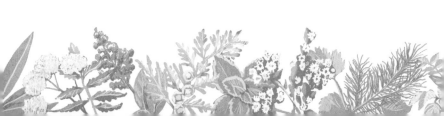

1. Stress
Round up the usual suspects here. Life throws us curve balls all the time: bad news, threatened redundancy, relationship worries, childcare issues, sickness, money problems, divorce, separation and breakups, difficult neighbors, work problems, arguments with friends, road rage, delayed travel, failed exams, challenging job interviews, even pandemics. These things can cause stress, and with too much cortisol and adrenalin in our blood streams, we tense up as we lie in bed trying to solve our problems in the middle of the night (things always seem worse then, in the dark, when you can't do much about them).

2. Sleep Disorders
Examples of sleep disorders include restless legs, itchy legs, and parasomnias such as night terrors, nightmares, sleepwalking, sleep talking, and sleep apnea (snoring). These can disrupt your sleep or even take you into dangerous situations (such as sleepwalking out of the house).

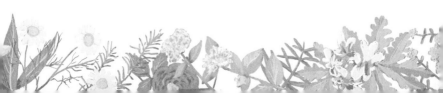

3. Physical Conditions

Illness and pain can cause insomnia, especially if you suffer from long-term chronic conditions, such as arthritis, high-blood pressure, or Parkinson's disease. You might have physical disruptions because of hormonal changes, such as during the menopause where the drop in estrogen and progesterone can cause night sweats. Pregnancy can keep women awake as it can be difficult to get comfortable, and many pregant women will have indigestion. Also, sleep seems to become rarer with age, so men as well as women may find themselves unable to sleep in their twilight years.

4. Mental Health Issues

Having a condition such as depression, anxiety, or ADHD (attention deficit hyperactivity disorder) can lead to lack of sleep. Ruminating on issues in the middle of the night, or having obsessive thoughts or repetitive ideas, as with OCD (obsessive compulsive disorder), can be exhausting and make it difficult to relax enough to fall asleep or to sleep well.

5. Medication

Sometimes the medication given for depression can actually keep you awake. People can have adverse reactions to antidepressants (there are many types) and over-the-counter drugs, which often have added caffeine and can affect sleep patterns. If you are trying to give up long-term use of antidepressants, this will change you neurologically, which can also affect sleep as you are adjusting to dropping off without them. A note: some people self-medicate with illegal drugs—not a great idea for a good night's sleep.

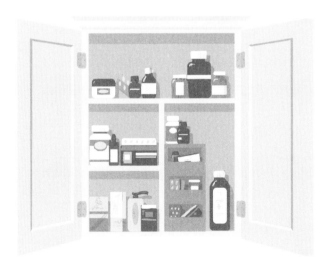

6. Food and Drink

Eating too much, too late can keep you awake. Fatty, fried, or spicy food can be difficult to digest, causing discomfort and making it hard to sleep. You might find food allergies keep you awake, too. Plus, too much alcohol or a nightcap may well wake you up during the night, despite the initial crashing out to sleep. Alcohol is dehydrating and makes you need to go to the bathroom more. Your deep REM sleep is interrupted, which is often why memory and dreams are impaired. Additionally, there is a hangover to deal with. Caffeine is added to a great deal of food and drink (sauces, ice cream, tea, coffee, fizzy drinks), and this can keep you wide-eyed in the night.

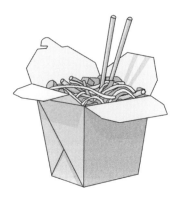

7. Your Environment

There are some key culprits that will keep you awake when you want to sleep:

Noise: from traffic, roads, public transit, music/sounds from neighbors, and gadgets in your room or house.

Light: from gadgets, lamps, televisions, streetlights.

Temperature: being too hot or too cold.

A snoring partner: unwittingly, sleep apnea can ruin a great night's sleep.

Toxins and chemical smells: from your own house or outside.

Unwanted pets on the bed: can make your bed too hot, hairy, smelly, or heavy.

Co-sleeping children: can be great for a while, especially if they have a nightmare or are scared, but it can interrupt your sleep to share your bed with children regularly.

BIG BAG OF WORRIES

If you can't sleep, it is a good idea to sit up or get up, have a warm (uncaffeinated) drink, and write down your worries. Write down absolutely everything, no matter how trivial, in a long list. I call this filling a big bag of worries. Try writing your list on paper, and at the end, scrunch it up and throw it in the trash before you go back to sleep. Or, you can fold it up and put it under your pillow and come back to it in the morning. It can make a great to-do list in the cold light of day, but you need a clear head, free of worries, to get a good night's sleep.

Practical exercise

DRAW YOUR FANTASY BED

Take some scrap paper, pens, pencils, or
crayons. Draw the kind of bed you'd love to
have just for fun—a real fantasy bed. Would it
be a giant four poster or a beautiful curvy
chaise longue? Maybe a bed shaped like a car or a
cool modern structure? A waterbed? Circular bed? Maybe a whole
room made of mattresses on the floor? Scribble away and come
up with something you'd really like to sprawl over or lounge on.

Practical
exercise

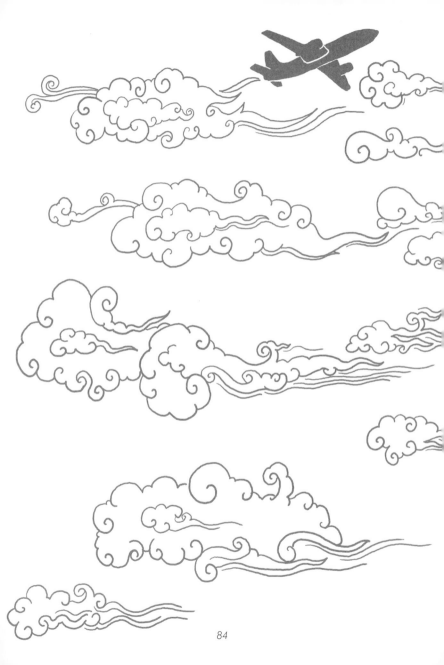

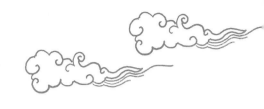

Jet lag

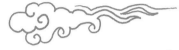

Mass long-distance airplane travel in the modern world means many people experience jet lag and consequential sleep disruption. The main issue with crossing time zones messes with our internal circadian rhythms, especially when traveling from west to east. It is hard to have to sleep when, internally, your body clock is telling you it is time to be awake. It takes about a day to recover from one hour of time difference, so traveling to the other side of the world—a twelve-hour time difference—can mean twelve days of waking up at three in the morning and feeling exhausted first thing.

Jet lag can be eased by taking melatonin and trying to enter into the time zone of the place you are visiting. It's best to stay up in the light and sleep in the dark, despite what your internal body clock is telling you to do. However, it is inevitable that there will be some insomniac nights and dozy days while your mind and body adjust to a new regimen.

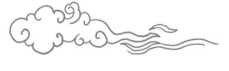
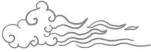

Creating the Right Environment for Sleep

Working out what makes you sleep better is an individual task. However, it is possible to do some basic things and create new, healthy habits so you can improve your sleep hygiene. After all, if you really want a good night's sleep, you can help yourself —this is where self-care really counts.

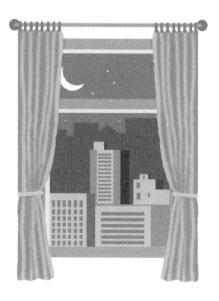

Bedroom

Your bedroom needs to be a calm place for sleep—and sex—but not set up for working, eating, gaming, or anything that interferes with your ability to slumber.

Temperature

Your bedroom needs to be cool at night: 60–65°F (16–18°C) is ideal. Overheated, airless rooms stop you being able to sleep well.

Décor

Make your bedroom sleep-inducing with soothing colors and fabrics. Some people like blues and greens, as they are calming. Others like warm pink, cream, brown, coral, terracotta tones. White gives a feeling of calm and space. Busy, crazy patterns and loud wallpapers might well keep you wide awake.

Declutter

An untidy, cluttered bedroom makes it difficult to rest and relax. If it is full of paperwork, newspapers, cans, dirty plates, bottles, and smelly socks, it is not very inviting for serene slumber.

Gadgets

A computer, laptop, or other gadgetery in your room including your cell phone, might lure you to use your screen late in the evening. This will wake your brain up and make sleep difficult. Try to stop using your devices for at least an hour before sleep. Limit blue light and use red light apps to make screens warmer, and you should sleep better. Turn gadgets off before you go to bed and try not to check them during the night.

Darkness

Light stimulates the brain to wake up, producing serotonin, so blackout blinds or lining for drapes and removing flashing LED lights are important for good-quality sleep.

Noise

Turn off bleeping gadgets and televisions, and wear earplugs if you need to blank out any external noise or a snoring partner.

Mattress

Your mattress needs to be firm but not too hard. It should be soft on your back and limbs but not squishy. If you have memory foam, a mixture with springs and other kinds of materials is best, as it can be too hot for good sleep. A mattress easily harbors dust mites and other bugs, so clean it regularly and replace it completely every eight years.

Sheets

Sheets need washing and changing weekly. Fresh, clean, even fragrant sheets can enhance a good night's sleep.

Pets

If you find having a dog or cat on your bed disturbs you, then keep them outside the room.

Children

If your children crawl into bed with you, make sure you take them back to their own bed and settle them back to sleep there, especially if you find it disturbs your sleep.

FOREST PATH

Visualization

This exercise is particularly good at bedtime
or if you wake during the night. Get comfortable
in bed, on a couch, on a mat, or on the floor. Put a
blanket or bed cover over you if you feel cool. Close your eyes and
breathe in and out slowly. Imagine in your mind's eye a beautiful
forest. Envision the canopy of trees overhead, the birdsong, the
small animals hopping, the light permeating through the boughs.
"See" all the colors of the leaves and trunks. Maybe there are
wildflowers or a squirrel running up a hole. Imagine the sun
dappling the forest floor as you walk down the path. See your feet,
one foot going in front of the other. You look up and see the forest
all around; you are alone and serene. Keep walking and looking at
your lovely surroundings. After a while, open your eyes and pause
for a second and see how you feel.

Physical Factors

Sleep is not only affected by environmental factors, such as light, noise, and temperature—it is also affected by what we do to ourselves. We might be experiencing stress, anxiety, and depression, or overwork and exhaustion, which interferes not only with getting to sleep but also staying asleep. It's common for us to adopt habits that seem to aid sleep, but in reality they actually stop our bodies from winding down. The good news is that the solution lies in our own hands: we can learn some new habits and adopt practices to help us experience good quality slumber.

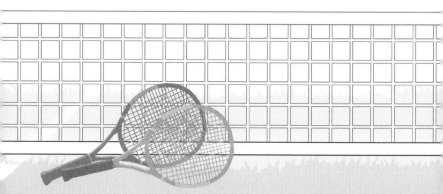

Exercise

Research shows that exercising for about thirty minutes during the day will improve your sleep. However, it is important not to do strenuous exercise after 9 p.m. at night as it will interfere with sleep as your bloodstream will be full of endorphins, which will keep you awake. Yoga, pilates, and stretching exercises can promote relaxation. It's a good idea to prepare for bed with neck and back stretches.

Food

The best foods to eat for a good night's sleep are eggs, fish, chicken, and nuts as they contain tryptophan, an amino acid, which is a building block for serotonin. Also, a couple of whole wheat crackers with peanut butter or cereal and milk before bed can help you sleep.

Alcohol

Drinking too much will keep you awake through dehydration, so drink plenty of water before bed and limit your intake. You should have at least one rest day a week so your liver can recover.

Drugs

Drugs may change your sleep/wake patterns as they are mind-altering. They also might include chemicals, which are damaging to your central nervous system, cause dehydration, make you eat erratically and late, and even trigger physical shock.

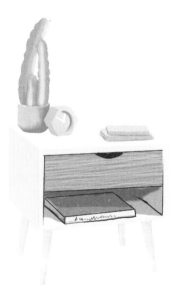

Caffeine

Limit caffeine or drink decaffeinated drinks in the run-up to bedtime. Try not to drink caffeine after 5 p.m. Also, a hot milky drink will induce sleepiness (but choose one with not too much chocolate, as that also contains caffeine).

Naps

Small sleeps or naps in the daytime are fine, just as long as they are short (only thirty minutes max) and before 3 p.m.. If they are longer and happen after that time, they tend to eat into the stage 3 REM sleep (see page 9) at night, which is the valuable deep sleep we all need. But a small nap can be a reallife saver, especially when under pressure.

Sex

Having a warm, satisfying cuddle or sex before bed can be a great sleep-inducer. Kissing releases oxytocin, which is a relaxing feel-good hormone (and also released when breastfeeding). If you are alone and sleepless, you can always pleasure yourself —enjoy your body and help yourself have a good night's sleep.

Breathing exercise

BUTEYKO BREATHING

Sit in bed with your mouth closed. Breathe through your nose naturally and easily for about thirty seconds, then breathe a bit more intentionally in and out through your nose, just once. Gently pinch your nose closed with your thumb and forefinger, keeping your mouth closed as well, until you feel you wish to breathe again. With your mouth still closed, release your nose, and take a deep breath in and out through your nose again. Stop, close your eyes, and relax.

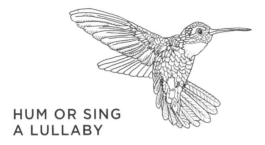

HUM OR SING
A LULLABY

You may well remember favorite lullabies from childhood or know them from singing to your children. Get comfortable and hum one or sing one to yourself. If you can't remember the words, just hum the tune and enjoy the feelings and sensations of making sound. This might bring back fond memories, or make you feel sad or nostalgic. Just let the memories and feelings wash over you, while you hum or sing quietly and relax.

Energizing
exercise

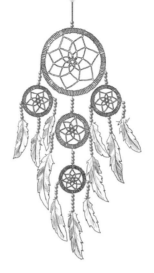

Your Mental State

When we head for bed, the biggest enemy against a good night's sleep is often lurking in our own heads. We may find that the minute we lie down our minds are racing, and we can't seem to stop thinking, causing anxiety to rise and our bodies to become tense. If we worry about how we will get to sleep, we tend to end up lying in bed, wide awake, worrying about not getting enough sleep or not waking up on time. Accumulated anxiety about being short of sleep, night after night, can also build into a phobia about sleeping. The good news is that there is plenty of help, research, and information to help you sleep. The first step is to acknowledge that your own mindset may be keeping you awake. Take a look at the following and see if you can adopt at least some of these proven good-sleep practices.

Meditation

Doing a simple meditation for five or ten minutes can help you get into a nice, calm, relaxed state for sleep (see page 25).

Creative Visualizations

Lying down and "seeing" a lovely scene in your mind, like a seashore or a beautiful meadow, can help you begin to chill out for slumber (see page 91).

Dump Your Worries

Writing down everything that is worrying you in a journal or notepad is a great way of emptying out your mind for sleep (see page 82).

Dream Journal

You might find yourself waking up with a nightmare or repetitive dream. It's a good idea to jot dreams down in the night (you can scribble in the dark in your notebook) or keep a dream journal in the morning. If you go for therapy, keeping a note of your dreams is very useful.

Talking

Sometimes in the night our worries can spill over, causing us to wake up feeling anxious, or prevent us from getting to sleep in the first place. It can feel like there will be a long, lonely, sleepless night ahead. If you need to talk, try speaking with your partner or spouse, or make an arrangement with a friend, so you can call or text them late. You can always call a helpline (see pages 159–160).

Sleep Aids

Not being able to drop off to sleep naturally can cause a great deal of distress and anxiety, which in turn affects sleep. When we are experiencing a prolonged time of stress, sleep can seem completely impossible. Luckily, there are many tried and tested remedies available to help us achieve quality sleep. Some are traditional remedies, some are based on alternative health practices, and some are science-based. Read on and see what might work for you.

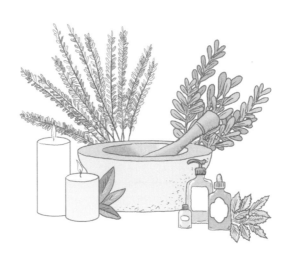

Breathing Apparatus

A breathing apparatus can be used to treat sleep apnea—a sleep disorder whereby your breathing is paused for up to ten seconds, ending in a snore. CPAP-masks can help reduce your snoring and increase your energy, even your libido, as your blood will be better oxygenated, and your sleep less interrupted. Sleep apnea can ruin relationships and can be disrupting for your own sleep and well-being—see your doctor or contact a sleep clinic (see pages 159-160) if you need help.

CBT-I (Cognitive Behavioral Therapy for Insomnia)

This is a form of CBT (cognitive behavioral therapy) that gives you progressive exercises designed to improve your sleep hygiene. Ask your doctor or research online for help. Make sure you go to a specialist or sleep clinic for advice.

Sleeping Pills

Most doctors are now reluctant to dish out sleeping pills, but they have their uses if you have experienced a trauma or a serious illness or operation. Only take under medical supervision. Also be aware that sleeping pills interfere with REM sleep and dreaming, so they are not a long-term solution. It is also important not to drink alcohol with them.

White Noise
This can help reduce outside noises or interfering sounds. You can find an app or use an air purifier or fan to make a consistent and soothing sound throughout the night.

Herbal Remedies
People have long used natural remedies for sleep, such as valerian root, magnesium (important for heart and brain function), passionflower, and glycine (an amino acid).

Herbal Teas
There are some specifically blended teas for inducing sleep; chamomile is relaxing, and rooibos is a good alternative to caffeinated tea.

Antihistamine
As allergies from pollen, dust, house dust mites, and pet dander can keep you awake if you are sneezing with rhinitis. You might find taking an antihistamine will help you sleep (don't take it as well as taking a sleep remedy based on histamine).

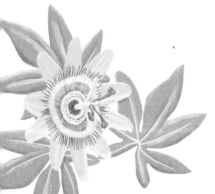

Melatonin

This hormone naturally rises in the evening and falls in the morning. It can improve sleep quality and seems to reduce the amount of time people need to fall asleep, plus gives them longer sleep. A dose of 3–10 milligrams can be taken before bedtime, but it should only be taken under the supervision of your doctor, pharmacist, or sleep clinic.

Fragrance

Lavender can put you in a relaxed state by reducing your heart rate and blood pressure, inducing a soporific state. You can use either lavender oil drops in a humidifier, scented candles, or roll-on scents. You could also place lavender bags under pillows, or buy lavender-filled pillows and eye masks.

Sleeping Preparations

Ask your pharmacist for sleep remedies based on histamines that help you get to sleep. You should check with your pharmacist or doctor as to whether you should use them or not as they can interfere with existing medication.

Natural Therapies

There any many holistic natural therapies—such as acupuncture, acupressure, shiatsu, reiki, aromatherapy, and reflexology—that can improve your sleep as they activate the body's natural healing mechanisms. This is a well-established mind-body-spirit approach to helping you sleep well.

CHAPTER FIVE

Sleep and Work

We generally spend more time at work than we do sleeping. How much we work, how many hours, where we work, what we do and with whom, plus the level of responsibility and control that we have, certainly affects our ability to sleep well. Worldwide, millions of working days are lost every year due to stress, depression, and anxiety. Workplace stress is one of the biggest destroyers of a sound night's sleep.

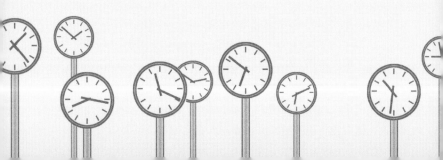

Reasons for Workplace Stress

Stress often happens when employees experience a high demand coupled with low control in the workplace. They can feel trapped in a high-pressure situation that they feel they have no power to change. Stress comes about because of feeling trapped between constant demand and the inability to meet it adequately.

People suffering from work-related stress, depression, and anxiety may experience:

Workload pressures

Tight deadlines

Feelings of having too much responsibility

Lack of managerial support

A sense of powerlessness to change their situation

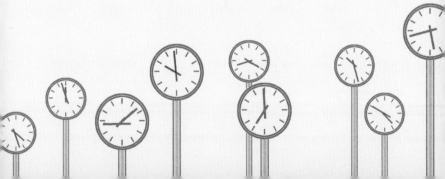

Stress and Sleep

Over time, a build-up of stress affects our ability to sleep, as we then have too much cortisol and adrenaline pumping in our bloodstreams. People feel "wired" by overload and caffeine. Then they drink alcohol to calm down, reaching for the beer, gin and tonic, or joint (or other mind-altering drugs) when getting home. These other substances, such as cocaine, also affect and interfere with sleep, along with junk food, eating too late, and staring at screens binge-watching, browsing, or chatting online.

Health Risks

Unfortunately, a stressful job plus poor sleep is a truly bad recipe for health and well-being and can lead to an early grave. People might use drink and drugs to fall asleep but then wake up at 4 a.m. to go to the bathroom and can't get back to sleep. They lie there in the dark, tossing and turning, while ruminating about unsolved problems and difficult conversations with colleagues. This can lead to hypertension and cardiovascular problems: it's a toxic cocktail for poor physical and mental health.

Double Shift

Not surprisingly, the primary caregivers of children or those of us who are caregivers for relatives tend to experience more stress than our partners, probably because they are working a "double shift"—first, a full- or part-time job and second, a night and weekend shift as a parent or caregiver. People who work in the education sector tend to be the most stressed, followed by those working in public administration and defense.

How Do You Relax?

Make a list of ten things you like to do to relax.
It might be gardening, walking, singing, dancing,
cleaning, swimming, running, watching TV. What do
you like to do? What really chills you out?

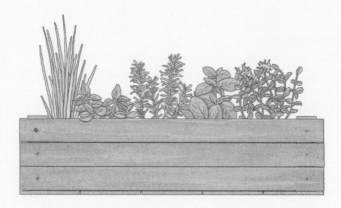

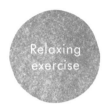

Relaxing exercise

HEAD-TO-TOE RELAXATION

Lie on your bed, couch, or the floor. Get comfortable and warm. Close your eyes. Take a deep breath. Exhale. Slacken your jaw and relax your shoulders into the floor; breathe in and out slowly. Feel your back supported by the floor, let it become heavier. Slacken your solar plexus. Let your arms sink into the floor, followed by your hips. Keep breathing in and out slowly. Let your buttocks sink into the floor, feel your thighs, calves, and ankles soften. Finally let your feet soften right down to your toes. Breathe in and out three times. Open your eyes.

Shift Work

An insidious by-product of the modern age is shift work. In the mid-twentieth century, people worked a typical nine-to-five schedule and clocked off at the end of the day. All of this changed with the demands of globalization and our 24/7 wakeful society. We have gotten used to increased productivity, constant international interconnection, and a lifestyle that never sleeps. Shift workers come in all shapes and sizes and are expected to perform around the clock and to order. Plus, with fewer full-time jobs and permanent contracts, many part-time workers are on an hourly rate without guaranteed shifts. They also often end up doing the most hazardous jobs.

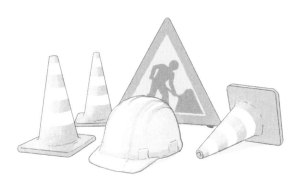

Shift-Work Disorder

Shift-work disorder is where your circadian rhythm has been disrupted. Having to work all night, or odd hours, and then trying to sleep in the daytime can lead to sleep disturbance. It can take time to adapt to a shift-work schedule, and for some professions and jobs schedules change all the time, making it very hard for the body and brain to adapt. Shift-work syndrome is a recognized sleep disorder and leads to people feeling excessively tired during waking hours. If you are in charge of a vehicle, you might be "drowsy driving." You will have a reduced performance at the tasks that you are in charge of, and this is a serious problem as shift workers are often employed in the most dangerous jobs. If your sleep is affected by night shifts, you might experience poor concentration, absenteeism, accidents, errors, or injuries.

YOUR WORK PATTERN

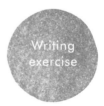

Writing exercise

Do you know exactly how many hours a day you work? Write down each day of the week and work out how long you were engaged in work-related tasks. Ask yourself: Do you work overtime, either paid or unpaid hours? How long do you commute for? How many hours are you engaged in work-based activities? How much work do you take home at night? Do you work weekends, and if so, for how long? Work out how many hours over a week you work exactly and balance this against how many hours a night you sleep on average.

The Effects of Overworking

Shift workers can also miss out on a range of social events, such as family parties and gatherings, holidays, vacations, special occasions, and play groups. It can also create emotional difficulties in personal relationships when one partner comes in late, as the other goes out: there is no time for conversation, and no relaxation time together, closeness, or sex. Being workers that pass in the night can have a seriously detrimental effect on intimacy and trust and can lead eventually to relationship breakdown.

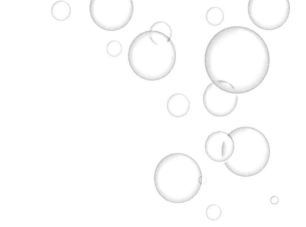

Calming exercise

BLOW BUBBLES

Find a couple of minutes to relax and de-stress.
Take a pot of bubbles and enjoy the experience
of blowing the soap solution through the plastic
ring. See how big a bubble you can blow. Lift
your arm with the bubble and send it up into
the air. Look at the colors, the shape of the
bubble, and watch it go. Enjoy it when it pops.
Blow several bubbles in a row, make a little
string of bubbles. You're never too old to enjoy
blowing bubbles. Have fun.

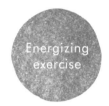

Energizing
exercise

NOTICE YOUR THOUGHTS

Take a moment away from your desk or whatever you
are doing. Sit or stand somewhere in private. Close your eyes for a
moment. Notice your thoughts. What is going on in your head?
What are you feeling in your stomach, your solar plexus? Where is
your attention? Notice any thoughts that float up or cross your
mind and let them go, like butterflies. Keep letting your thoughts
float through your head, but don't linger on them or worry about
them—just let them go. Thought after thought, butterfly after
butterfly. Watch them fly away.

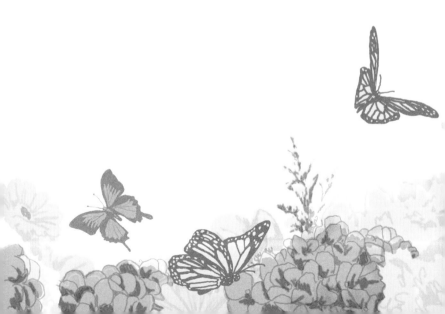

Physiological Effects of Shift Work

Research shows that shift workers are also at increased risk of gastrointestinal diseases, as well as cardiovascular disease. Again, this is due to the disruption of the circadian rhythm, the lack of light, or strange eating and drinking patterns than can develop around work. Night shifts and shift work has been linked to obesity, as you burn fewer calories at night and sleep in the day when you would be burning the most.

Microsleeps

As people feel a sleep debt due to sleep deprivation, they might have microsleeps during the day. This is when people fall asleep for a few seconds. One of the dangers of this involuntary behavior is that they might be at the wheel, using machinery, or looking after children when they blank out.

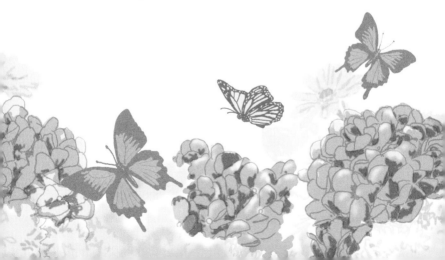

How Do You Stay Awake?

We all have our favorite tricks and ways of staying awake. What do you do? Get up and walk around? Go outside into the light? Throw the windows open to let fresh air in? Run? Dance? How do you pep yourself up? A can of cola? Phoning a friend? Jot down what you do and what you would like to do. What works best for you?

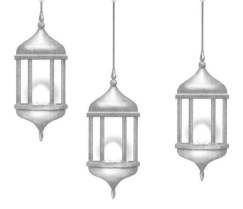

Staying Alert on a Night Shift

A thoughtful employer would enable the following to happen so that their employees ameliorate the impact of night-shift disorders. However, you need to be aware of what you need to do to help yourself:

Avoid driving due to the danger of microsleeping or nodding off.

Avoid extended work hours.

Take short naps (if possible) during a shift to keep going.

Work with others to keep alert.

Drink caffeine to keep awake.

Don't leave tedious or boring tasks until the end of a night shift —it's hard to keep awake between 4 and 5 a.m.

Collaborate with colleagues to solve problems.

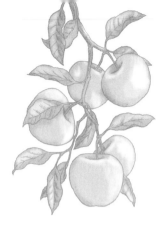

TWO-FRUIT JUGGLE

Try this during a break or at the end of a shift. Take two oranges, two apples, or two satsumas. Put one fruit in each hand. Turn your hands palm upward, with the heel of your hands together. Throw one fruit up in the air (not too far) with your right hand. Catch it with your left at waist height, pass it from your left to your right, then throw it straight up into the air with your right. Catch it with your left. Repeat. This is a basic two-fruit juggle. As you get faster, juggling two fruits in the air, add in the third fruit if you want more of a challenge. See if you can do it. The trick is to have one fruit in the air, traveling from your right hand to your left hand. One fruit goes up in the air, while there is still one in your left hand, which is tossed to the right and then thrown up in the air. And so on. It's tricky but but fun. You can also eat the fruit as a reward.

Relaxing exercise

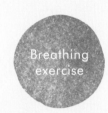

Breathing exercise

4-7-8 BREATHING TECHNIQUE

This exercise was developed by Dr. Andrew Weil as a variation of pranayama, an ancient yogic technic that aids relaxation as it replenishes the body with oxygen. Sit or lie comfortably in your bedroom or a private space. Allow your lips to part gently. Exhale completely, making a breathy "whoosh" sound as you do it. Press your lips together as you inhale silently through your nose for a count of four seconds. Hold your breath for a count of seven seconds. Exhale for a full eight seconds, making a whooshing sound throughout. Repeat four times.

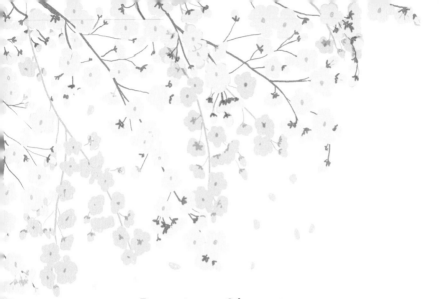

Daytime Sleeping

Although a lot of people will still have some kind of traditional work schedule (albeit it could be odd hours and late nights), the really tough issue is learning to sleep through the daytime. This is tough on many people, as your body and mind may never fully adapt to the regime. However, there are some things you can do to help yourself adjust.

Golden Hour

The "golden hour" is the wind-down time after a night shift or late shift and before going to bed. Try these tips to help you sleep during the daytime:

If your shift finishes during the daytime, wear sunglasses to block out the light.

Avoid caffeine and alcohol.

Have a warm bath or shower to calm down.

Do some gentle physical activity, such as yoga or pilates.

Have sex or pleasure yourself to feel more relaxed.

Meditate or use creative visualization.

Do the 4-7-8 Breathing exercise (see page 119).

Listen to calming music or white noise to drop off.

Wear an eye mask to bed or use blackout blinds.

Have earplugs on hand to fend off any noise disturbance from family and street life.

Write down any nagging issues in your Big Bag of Worries (see page 82) to be dealt with later.

CHAPTER SIX

Sleep and Relationships

How well we enjoy sleeping in the same space as our partners really matters. Sharing a bed with your partner or spouse is crucial for the well-being and healthy maintenance of any loving relationship. However, when sleep is not going well for one of the bedfellows, there can be a serious impact on a couple's happiness and life. Although we need at least eight hours sleep a night, many of us are getting by on only about six hours or less. So, if one of you is not sleeping well together, due to insomnia, shift work, or personal lifestyle habits, it will certainly impact your relationship.

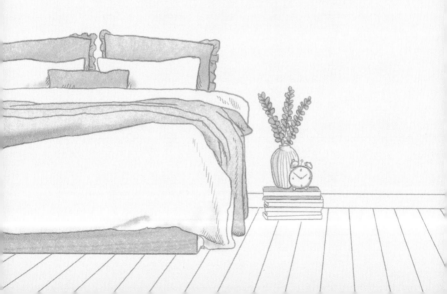

Sleep Deprivation Arguments

When we are sleep-deprived, the body and brain is already under stress. This means our bloodstreams are full of the fight, flight or freeze biochemicals, such as adrenalin or cortisol. Too much of these substances can make us very hyped-up. The amygdala in the brain is thrown out of kilter and this upsets our emotional balance. A sleep-deprived partner may well be snappy and overreactive as they become inflamed over things that they would usually take comfortably in their stride. Small things can blow out of all proportion into big conflicts, and irritability can lead to arguments.

Physiological Issues

Even having just one or two nights of lousy sleep can lead to heated arguments, according to research by Ohio State University (Wilson et al, 2017). In a study involving forty-three couples, arguments occurred between sleep-deprived couples concerning money, in-laws, and communication. They also measured levels of markers, such as the proteins IL-6 and TNF-alpha, whose rise can trigger the onset of serious chronic diseases, such as diabetes. It was the stress of a nasty fight that led to the onset of these markers in the blood. Sleep deprivation can also lead to physiological difficulties as it raises levels of inflammation in the body and creates "stressors." Apart from simply feeling tired and becoming exhausted, your immune system may be seriously challenged, leading to more colds and flu. Over time you might develop diabetes, cardiovascular disease, even cancer.

Keeping Things Calm

If one partner sleeps badly, a well-rested companion might be able to withstand the storm. Someone has to stay calm, after all. However, the worst-case scenario is when both people are struggling with lack of sleep, as in the early days, weeks, and months of parenthood. These times can be very trying, especially if one or both partners are also working. Other difficult times might be during a crisis, trauma, or illness.

Long-term sleep deprivation over weeks or months can lead to depression, anxiety, and even aggression. A tired partner can be irritable, anxious, and abrupt; two tired partners can be emotionally apocalyptic and physiologically damaging. It's very tempting, but one of the most aggravating things you can say to a tired and irritable partner is *"calm down."* It's probably not a good idea to say this as it may make things worse.

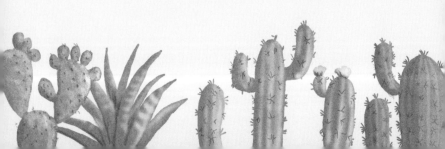

PAUSE AN ARGUMENT

Calming
exercise

When you are irritated or angered by your
partner, it is all too easy to get into a tit-for-tat
circular argument. It is also tempting to escalate the
argument, especially if you both feel tired and annoyed by a bad
night's sleep. A helpful tip is to say, as lightly as you can, without
blaming anyone, *"Let's pause here,"* and agree to come back to the
conversation at another time. Arguments can often go round and
round repetitively, and go nowhere. Each partner just ends up even
more furious, frustrated, and entrenched with the other. It's
important to stop things before they go too far and before you do
or say anything you may regret later. Pausing means you break the
cycle of aggression.

Go away from your partner and breathe. Slow, deep, inhale, exhale.
Count to ten, then count from ten back to one. Take time away
from each other to cool down. If you acknowledge to yourself you
are tired, then you can say to your partner, when you return, *"Let's
talk about this after we've had some sleep."* It's a way of saying,
"calm down," without being patronizing, while acknowledging that
your lack of good-quality slumber has something to do with your
mood. Sleep separately if you are still feeling annoyed and then
sort things out in the clear light of day.

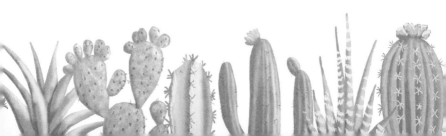

No Sex, We're Sleep-Deprived

When you don't feel your best physically due to poor
sleep, this can reduce your libido and lead to an unsatisfying
sex life with your partner. It might even lead to no sex at all.
Sadly, this can exacerbate any deep seated emotional and
relationship problems you already have as a couple. Lack of sex
is also a sign that things are not really working well between
you emotionally, and lack of sleep just makes it all
feel so much worse.

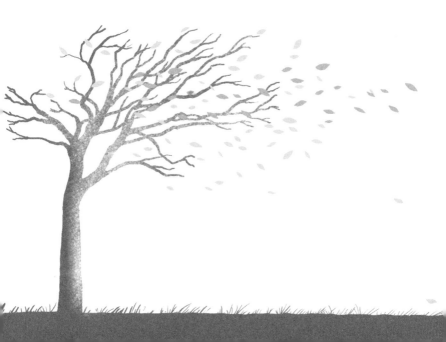

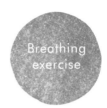

Breathing exercise

BHRAMARI PRANAYAMA BREATHING EXERCISE

This exercise quickly reduces your heart rate and calms your breathing. It is good for preparing your body for sleep. Find a private space and get comfortable on a chair or couch. Close your eyes and breathe deeply, in and out. Keep breathing and cover your ears with your hands. Place each index finger above each eyebrow and place the rest of your fingers over your eyes. With your little fingers flat against your face, press the sides of your nose, and put your mental focus on your brow area as you breathe in and out. Keep your mouth closed and breathe out slowly through your nose, making a humming "om" sound. If you have time, repeat three or five times before bed.

Sleep Apnea

When a partner snores, this can cause sleep deprivation in the other partner. People who live with snorers and who are woken up three times a night for about ten minutes each time themselves can experience sleep disorders as a consequence. This is a level of insomnia that can lead to lower relationship satisfaction and impaired functioning the next day. Snoring can make frustrated and weary couples move into separate bedrooms, which is not ideal for marital harmony (although it works well for some). However, it can be a thin end of the wedge toward separation and divorce if a couple is not communicating well and is unable to maintain compassion, intimacy, and sex.

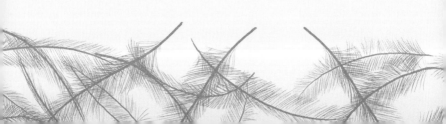

RELAXING HIP POSE

This is a good exercise to do before bed as it is relaxing and helps you flex your muscles and tend to your back. It is especially good if you have spent much of the day sitting at a desk or driving. Find a quiet, comfortable floor or bed. You need a couple of cushions or pillows, or you could roll up a blanket or coat and put it under your back for comfort.

Sit on the floor and bring the soles of your feet together. Put your arms behind you and lean back on your hands, palms down. Lean back gently onto the floor, with your back, neck, and head now on the floor. Bring your arms to either side of you on the floor, palms up, slightly away from your sides. With your feet still together, let your knees fall gradually to either side of your body, so you have an open lap. Feel your lower back pressing gently against the floor as you press your feet together. Hold this pose for two minutes. Relax and bring your knees back up to the center. Repeat three times.

Relaxing exercise

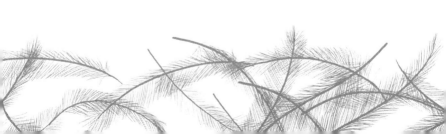

Attraction and Sleep

Interestingly, if you don't sleep well you may actually put your partner off finding you sexually attractive. In 2010, researchers in Sweden found that well-rested people actually appear more attractive to others. People who were sleep-deprived were rated less attractive and unhealthy-looking, not very amusing, witty, or flirtatious. A 2015 study by David A. Kalmbach and other researchers showed that people who have enough sleep seem to be more sexually responsive. In particular, women who sleep well are more arousable genitally than those with shorter sleep patterns. Overall, sleep deprivation not only increases conflict but also reduces the satisfaction that we get from of our sex lives—so getting enough sleep is certainly important for couples.

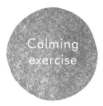

Calming exercise

SOOTHING NIGHTTIME DRINK

If you are finding it hard to sleep or want a warm drink before bedtime, try this. Take a mug of milk, or oat or almond milk, and warm it gently. Add two teaspoons of hot chocolate and stir. Heat it to your preferred temperature and sprinkle with cinnamon. Dunk something tasty, like oat or ginger cookies, into it to make a good soothing night-time snack. Cow's milk has an amino acid called tryptophan in it, which can help you drift off to sleep.

Making Decisions

When one or both partners are tired, it is very difficult to discuss contentious issues and make tough decisions rationally. Sleep deprivation interferes with cognitive function, and people find it hard to listen to each other and remember what has been said. As partners might feel sensitive and overreactive, they can also feel more rejected if they feel the other person is not listening or does not agree with them. A small misinterpreted issue can develop into a full-blown misunderstanding because one or both partners are not able to pay attention to what is being communicated. Couples often try and discuss things in a rush when they are going out the door in the morning, or late at night after a few drinks: this can lead to full-scale screaming matches, which is never a good idea.

MINDFUL SHOWER OR BATH

Calming exercise

Make time for a luxury bath or shower before bed. Having a nice, relaxing bath is one of those things that will help with sleep. Either stand under the shower soaping yourself with your favorite shower gel, or pour some lovely bubble bath into your tub. Spend time just feeling the warm soapy water on your skin and the heat pervade your bones and body. Enjoy savoring the aromas and the sensation of washing your skin with soap, flannel cloth, or sponge. Try to do this in silence, without music, radio, or podcasts, and just stay with the bodily sensations. Close your eyes for a few moments as you soap yourself and think *"All is well."* Repeat this as you breathe in and out slowly, three times. Finish your ablutions and wrap yourself up in a lovely warm towel. A variation on this exercise involves including your partner, washing each other slowly or sharing a nice soak in the tub, which can be fun before bed.

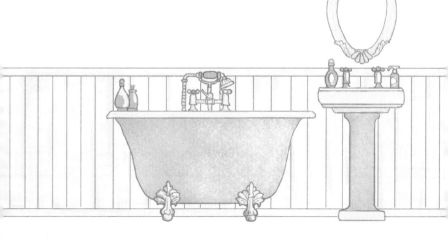

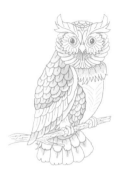

Owls and Larks

Our particular chronotypes can determine whether we are night owls or morning larks. Night owls tend to wake later in the morning, then have a second wind in the evening. Morning larks tend to wake early but are ready to go to bed at 10 p.m. If partners are opposite chronotypes, this can cause a great deal of domestic disharmony. In order to be happy together, couples need to learn to accommodate each other's inherent differences. It is not a good idea to try and change each other; rather, it is important to understand that there are different rhythms to life. Owls can learn to make love in the morning, sometimes, and larks can decide to stay up for special events. A little thoughtful accommodation can go a long way. Plus, as people move into midlife and beyond, these rhythms may be a little more flexible, so couples can meet halfway, timewise.

WHICH ARE YOU?

Ask yourself the following questions. You could also do this with your partner:

1. Do you like getting up early to see the dew on the leaves or even the dawn?

2. Are you happier seeing the moon and stars at night, and watching the night sky?

3. Do you find it hard to stay awake and focus after about 10 p.m.?

4. Do you seem to get a second wind around 10 p.m. and can stay awake into the early hours?

If you answered "yes" to questions one and three, you are a lark, and if you answered "yes" to questions two and four, you are an owl. Interestingly, larks are slightly more adaptable than owls and can usually train themselves to stay up a bit later, if they want to. Owls are not lazy; they just have a different circadian rhythm to larks.

Practical exercise

Mirror Image Relationships

Psychologists find that people often choose partners who have similar traits to themselves. These may be physical traits, such as the distance between the eyes, or personality traits. Ideally, if two similar people choose each other—like two owls or two larks— they will mirror each other and probably find it easier to live with each other. Choosing a partner with similar features is called assortative mating and is evident throughout the animal kingdom.

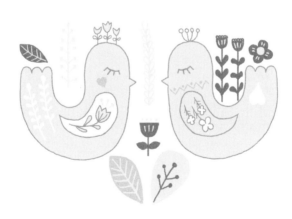

NIGHTY-NIGHT NECK STRETCH

Before you go to bed, try this exercise. It's a good way of ironing out all the stresses and creases from the day before you try to get to sleep. Find a quiet space to stand, possibly in your bedroom in your night clothes, underwear, or even naked, if you fancy it. Stand up straight, with your knees soft. Drop your chin down to your chest and hold for five breaths. Bring your head back up to the center, then let it fall back for five breaths. Repeat this five times, going as slowly as you can, blowing a deep breath out as you drop your chin, and breathing in as you raise it. Don't worry if you hear some clicks and cracks from your vertebrae as you do, as that's normal.

Relaxing exercise

CHAPTER SEVEN

Sleep and Children

Mention sleep to most parents and they will probably groan, roll their eyes, then regale you with tales of sleepless nights spent rocking their children. Or grimace as they remember all those hours of nighttime diaper changing, breastfeeding until dawn, or dealing with colic. Indeed, they might well have something to moan about, as researchers have found that parents lose 350 hours of sleep during the first year after birth. They also lose a staggering 645 hours of sleep in raising a child from infancy to the end of their offspring's eighteenth year.

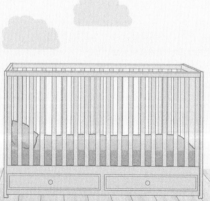

Parental Sleep Deprivation

One or two children can mean a huge amount of nocturnal slumber time lost for parents. Overall, sleep deprivation goes on for about six years, and many parents feel they never really have a good night's sleep again as parental concern continues as the children grow. What's more, mothers tend to lose more sleep than fathers, especially in the first three months of a baby's life.

New Parents and Sleep

When a couple have a baby, there will be a lot to think about, and sleep can be a major preoccupation. We know that adults need something like seven to nine hours sleep a night, yet a newborn is going to reduce the number of hours slept because parents needing and wanting to meet its needs. A 2013 study called "The Sleep-Time Cost of Parenting" showed that 41 percent of new parents sleep less than seven hours a night during the first year. Some people need more sleep than others, while others are more flexible. This can be due to individual personality and chronotype. However, a new breastfeeding mother (or bottlefeeding parent) will be tied to their baby's needs. Although this can be very satisfying and necessary, it can also really destroy a good night's sleep.

Side Effects

There can be side effects with sleep depreviation, as tired parents make cranky parents. New parents have shorter sleep, interrupted sleep, and disrupted REM sleep. Sleep supports good physical and mental health, and new parents are usually sleep-deprived just at the point where they need it the most.

Negative Feelings

Not surprisingly, many relationships break down during
the first year after a baby comes along due to the stress of
putting a newborn's needs, before the needs (and sleep time) of
each partner. Studies have found that sleep-deprived parents
can feel negatively toward their own children. They can also
end up feeling resentful about their parental role. Plus, parents
who are working can end up being unproductive, or even
absent, because they are too tired to function.

SMALL SKETCH

Practical exercise

This exercise is great for helping you to relax and unwind after a busy day. Take a piece of a paper and a pen, and look at a small object on your desk or in your house. It could be a stone, an ornament, a flower, or a utensil. Put it on a table and look at it for a minute, then take your pen and draw it. Don't hold back—just enjoy feeling your pen flow over the paper. Look hard at the object and follow its lines, then sit back and enjoy your work.

SHOULDER ROLL

Relaxing exercise

Find a private or quiet space and stand with your feet hip-width apart. Raise your shoulders up to your ears, squeeze them together, then drop them down again. Do this three times. Roll one shoulder up and back, then the other. Do this slowly, feeling the ligaments and muscles release. Roll each shoulder three times on each side.

Co-Sleeping and Bedsharing

One solution to the first year of sleep deprivation during an infant's life is co-sleeping. In some cultures, it is accepted that a baby will share a parent's bed for ease of breastfeeding and for maternal comfort. While in India 85 percent of preschoolers sleep with their parents, this is generally less acceptable in other cultures. Some people like to put the baby next to the parental bed in a crib for easy access, while others prefer the baby to be sleeping in their own cot right from the start. If you do decide to co-sleep, always follow the latest safety advice.

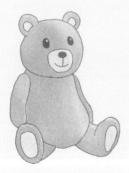

TWO-MINUTE RELAXATION

Relaxing
exercise

Set your timer and find a quiet space—a couch, a bed, or the floor. Put something over your eyes, like a sweater or eye mask. Put in earplugs, if you need them. Lie on your back and stretch out. Make sure your head is supported. Close your eyes. Widen your jaw as if to yawn, to relax your face. Let yourself fall into the couch, bed, or floor. Relax yourself from head to toe, slowly imagining each part of your body becoming soft and heavy. Keep your mind on your body, focusing on each part in turn, and breathing steadily and deeply as you go. Allow yourself to relax until your timer goes off.

ALTERNATE NASAL BREATHING

This stress-reducing exercise, also called Shodhana Pranayama, is good before bed. Sit with your legs crossed or with your back supported against a wall in a sitting position. Place your left hand on your knee and your right thumb against your nose. Exhale fully and then close the right nostril with your thumb. Open your right nostril and exhale, while closing the left with your right index finger. Continue this rotation, alternating nostrils. Rest for a minute and notice how you feel afterward.

Breathing
exercise

Children's Sleep Deprivation

When children don't get enough sleep, it can have side effects on their health and well-being. High levels of the hormones ghrelin and leptin are produced in sleep-imbalanced children, which can cause them to feeling hungry even when they are full. This can lead to snacking on fatty, sugary, or salty foods, which increases the risk of obesity. Also, children sent to bed with a screen to help them sleep can actually be counter productive, as the screen will make falling asleep more difficult. Up until recently, melatonin was only prescribed to the over 55s, but now it is being given to sleep-deprived children, despite not knowing the long-term side effects. Limiting screens in the first place is a better path for parents to follow, if at all possible.

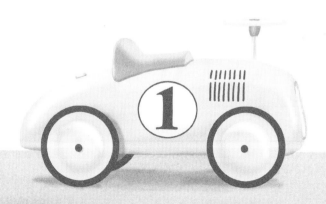

How Much Sleep Do Children Need?

Children of different ages require different amounts of sleep. Most paediatricians recommend the following for good sleep hygiene:

Babies, 4–12 months: 12–16 hours, including naps

Toddlers, 1–2 years: 11–14 hours, including naps

Children, 3–5 years: 10–13 hours, including naps

Children, 6–12 years: 9–12 hours

Teenagers, 13–18 years: 8–10 hours

Practical exercise

DOWNLOAD THEIR WORRIES

If your child seems anxious at bedtime, you could turn this exercise into a game. Draw a big bag and ask them to color it in; then at bedtime you or your child can write down their worries onto small pieces of paper and put them into the "bag." As children grow, it's a good idea to teach them they can help themselves to sleep by downloading their worries at night. Children won't necessarily tell you what's bothering them if you ask directly, but they might tell you this way if it's a bit of a game. It should also relieve them of their worries so they can sleep better.

Bedtime Routines

Younger children in particular will benefit from a calm, soothing bedtime routine, such as a warm, milky drink followed by a bath and a story. Try not to let children watch screens for at least an hour before bedtime and ensure that their bedroom is cool, well-ventilated, and dark (use a blackout curtain if necessary as darkness blocks serotonin and increases melatonin). Use a gentle night-light, music box, or something similar as a soother if a child finds it hard to get to sleep. You can get white noise apps or apps which replicate the sound of being inside the mother's abdomen, if a child finds it hard to get to sleep. Put older children's cell phones and devices in a secure box outside of the bedroom for the night and explain why. Also ensure that children don't have food or fizzy drinks in bedrooms—water only—and that pets are kept out.

MAKE A BEDTIME AROMA

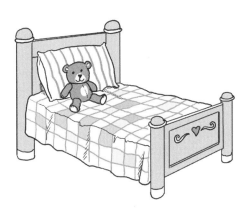

Practical
exercise

Aromatherapy diffusers are available online or
from most health-food stores, and are a great way
to create a calming aroma in a child's bedroom. First
ensure the diffuser is positioned safely out of the child's reach,
then add two or three drops of pure lavender, sweet basil, and
jasmine oils to the water. Put this on for about thirty minutes
before bedtime to enhance the calming atmosphere. Remember to
remove the diffuser before the child goes to bed.

CHAPTER EIGHT

Good Sleep for Life

Imagine getting into bed at night, tired and
sleepy, sinking into the mattress, snuggling under the duvet,
and waking up a full eight hours later, completely refreshed and
ready for the day ahead. Sounds a bit like a fairytale, but this
kind of sleep used to be possible when the world was slower,
less tech-obsessed, quieter, and less demanding. It wasn't
perfect for everyone, obviously, but people were not as
overstimulated as we seem to be today. The onus on each and
every one of us in the twenty-first century and beyond is to learn
how to wind down and look after ourselves enough to get a
good, replenishing night's sleep.

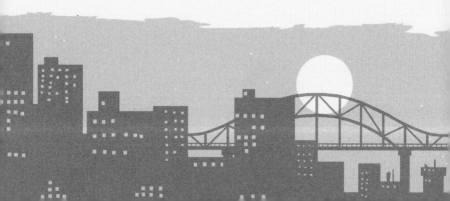

Self-Care for Sleep

To this end, knowing yourself is essential. Understanding how much sleep you need, whether you benefit from naps and what conditions you personally need for a decent slumber is crucial. It is also important to know which of your daily habits and behaviors are getting in the way of you falling or staying asleep. The way we live now has, in so many ways, caused us to forget that we are animals at heart, living with our individual circadian rhythms and being governed by the light, the dark, and even the moon.

It's also important to know whether you are a morning lark or night owl (see pages 134–135) so that you understand the optimal times of day that work for you. Knowing your own particular daily rhythms can help you choose the right work for you, based on whether you can get up early or stay up late. It can also help you work out which kind of chronotype partner will work for you best—are you both night owls, or is the issue of bedtime always going to be contentious, as one of you wants to nod off at 10 p.m. just when the other is getting a second wind?

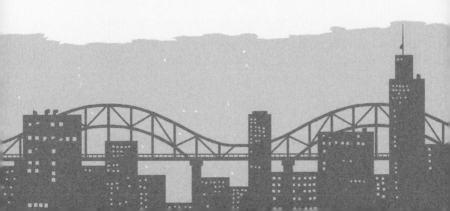

Attend to Yourself to Improve Your Sleep

Developing an attitude with self-care at the core means looking after yourself and your health. It means seeing a doctor when you need to or getting treatment for an injury or illness. It also means taking proactive care of your body and well-being. This is about valuing yourself and treating yourself like the precious being that you are. When you suffer in silence, or you ignore symptoms or tough out injuries, you are being thoughtless toward yourself.

A lack of self-care means a lack of compassion toward yourself. If you can't be compassionate toward yourself, then it will be hard to be kind to others. So it's worth taking time to look after yourself and think about how you live your life and how it affects your sleep. Without good sleep, both your mental and physical health will suffer. If you are not well, any dependents will suffer, and you won't be able to live your life to the full. It is an area really worth attending to for your own benefit and others.

SLEEP JOURNAL

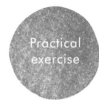

This journal only takes a few minutes to fill in, but is useful in understanding more about yourself, your habits, and your circadian rhythms. Keep a journal for a couple of weeks to give yourself a true picture of your sleep needs. Each day note down:

What time you went to bed

What time you woke up

How you felt on waking

How many times you woke during the night and the reasons

How many times today you felt sleepy

Anything else that may affect your sleep, such as monthly cycle, shift work, or travel

Number of caffeinated drinks consumed and time of last drink

Number of alcoholic drinks consumed and time of last drink

Foods eaten and time of last meal/snack

Exercise—what, when, and for how long

Screen use—what, when, and for how long

Naps—when and for how long

Medications—what taken and when

Sleep environment and bedtime routine

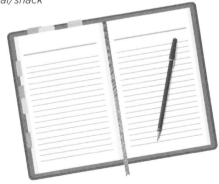

Twelve Steps to a Good Night's Sleep

While everyone is different, there are some basic principles for good sleep hygiene that have been worked out by experts. Following most, if not all of these steps, will help you get some good-quality shut-eye.

1. Go to bed and get up at the same time each day, if you possibly can. Sleeping late on the weekends won't necessarily pay off your sleep debt of too many late nights. Set an alarm for the same time every day and stick to it as much as you can.

2. Watch your caffeine intake over the course of the day and remember that coffee has a higher proportion of caffeine per cup than tea (almost double). Only drink caffeinated drinks up until around 5 or 6 p.m. Note that caffeine also lurks in fizzy drinks, ice cream, cakes, chocolate bars, and some medication.

3. Avoid too much alcohol, particularly a nightcap, as it will probably disturb your sleep. It will interfere with valuable REM sleep, dehydrate you, and make you get up in the night for the bathroom. You also might have a hangover, which means being dehydrated and less productive the next day. Drink alcohol within the recommended limits and have at least two alcohol-free days to catch up on quality sleep.

4. Exercise will help you sleep, but don't do a vigorous workout after 9 p.m. at night. This will keep you awake and buzzing. Instead try gentle stretches, yoga, or pilates at bedtime to wind down.

5. Don't eat large meals last thing, especially after drinking alcohol. Eating fatty, spicy, calorie-laden food late at night can lead to indigestion, which will interfere with sleep. Some foods, such as milk and cereal, crackers and peanut butter, or cheese, are sleep-inducing, Eat only as a light snack.

6. If you nap, only nap up until 3 p.m., or it will interfere with your deep stage 3 sleep (see page 9), which is important for memory retention and rejuvenation. Also, you may find it harder to drop off at night. Limit any naps to forty minutes.

7. Try not to take medicines that delay your sleep—some prescribed and over-the-counter preparations will wire you up (like additives in cough medicines, for instance). Read labels carefully and notice what disturbs your sleep. Talk to your pharmacist or doctor if you are concerned.

8. A hot, relaxing bath before bed will help you sleep. Using a lavender, chamomile, or jasmine perfumed bubble bath by candlelight should help you really nod off in bed.

9. Make sure your room is a dedicated bedroom, if possible. Remove office equipment, flashing LED lights, or gadgets (and block blue light for an hour before bedtime). Make it dark with blackout blinds or drapes to ensure a good sleep. Have a good mattress, pillow, and bedding. Keep your bedroom decluttered, cool, and calm.

10. Get some natural light on your body in the morning, as soon as possible. Go out for a short walk into in the yard, or on your balcony. Get out of your office and away from your desk at lunchtime, too. Light activates serotonin and helps you feel awake. It also helps regulate your inner body clock.

11. Meditate before bed, if you can, for five or ten minutes. Or do a creative visualization of walking by the sea, in the mountains, or through a lovely meadow (see page 91). Calm your mind down with benign visions of nature.

12. Dump your concerns into your Big Bag of Worries (see page 82) or on paper. If you can't get to sleep after twenty minutes, get up and go and do something else, like reading, having a warm drink, doing a crossword, or even writing down more worries. Go back to bed when you begin to feel a bit drowsy.

Being Positive about Sleep

It is possible to change our attitudes toward our ability to sleep well. We often feed ourselves negative ideas and they become beliefs, such as *"I am a bad sleeper"* or *"I'll never get a good night's sleep."* As with most things, if you begin to train your mind to think more positively, it will help you approach your sleeping in a different way. Don't think you are stuck with bad sleep patterns for life; you can take charge and believe you can do something about it.

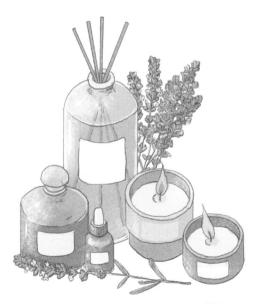

Making the Change

Improving our sleep by getting enough hours in the right conditions is completely possible, even in our modern, fast-moving world. The most important step is to decide to help yourself sleep better and then put the suggestions in this book into practice.

We each need to look at our physical needs, our environment, and our psychological mindset. If you want a better night's sleep—and to keep it a regular experience—then you can. However, it will take some effort to look at how you treat your body, what kind of sleep environment you have created, and to learn some simple techniques to calm your mind.

The good news is there are plenty of apps to help and also lots of resources out there that are easily accessible, such as earplugs and lavender oil, eye masks and calming music and simple meditation and massage. Take charge of your own sleep needs, and you will definitely see the benefits.

I CAN SLEEP

Try planting these positive ideas in your mind and they'll gradually sink in. Say them to yourself as a mantra as you are settling down for the night:
"*I can easily get to sleep*".
"*I can sleep all night through*".
"*I'm snug as a bug in a rug.*"
"*I am safe, relaxed, and drifting off to sleep.*"

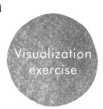
Visualization exercise

Resources

Apps
Calm
Headspace
The Mindfulness App
Stop, Breathe & Think

Psychological Help
Mental Health America
www.mhanational.org/get-involved/contact-us

Warmline
www.warmline.org

National Alliance on Mental Illness
www.nami.org

Anxiety and Depression Association of America (ADAA)
www.adaa.org

The Trevor Project
www.thetrevorproject.org

Depression and Bipolar Support Alliance
www.dbsalliance.org

National Eating Disorder Association
www.nationaleatingdisorders.org

Meditation/Mindfulness
Be Mindful
www.bemindful.co.uk

Breathworks
www.breathworks-mindfulness.org.uk

Mind
www.mind.org.uk

Mindful
www.mindful.org

Samaritans
www.samaritans.org

Sleep

American Sleep Apnea Association
www.sleepapnea.org

Circadian Sleep Disorders Network
www.circadiansleepdisorders.org

Restless Legs Syndrome Foundation
www.rls.org

Narcolepsy Network
www.narcolepsynetwork.org

American Sleep Association
www.sleepassociation.org

Confidence

The Dove Self-Esteem Project
www.dove.com/us/en/dove-self-esteem-project.html

The Cybersmile Project
www.cybersmile.org

OneLove
www.joinonelove.org

Loveisrespect
www.loveisrespect.org

Books

The Mindfulness Journal by Corinne Sweet

The Anxiety Journal by Corinne Sweet

Full Catastrophe Living: How to Cope With Stress, Pain, and Illness Using Mindfulness by Jon Kabat-Zinn

About the Author

Corinne Sweet is an author, psychotherapist, psychologist, and broadcaster. She is the author of several popular psychology bestsellers, such as *Change Your Life with CBT*, *The Anxiety Journal*, *The Mindfulness Journal*, *How to Say No*, *Overcoming Addiction*, and *Stop Fighting About Money*. Corinne trained on BBC Radio 4's *Woman's Hour* and was a magazine and newspaper advice columnist and a *Big Brother* psychologist. She appears regularly on TV and radio, collaborating frequently with BBC Breakfast and BBC Radio Scotland. Corinne blogs regularly at www.corinnesweet.com.

Corinne is a psychotherapist at City Therapy Rooms (www.citytherapyrooms.co.uk) and Barnsbury Therapy Rooms (www.barnsburytherapyrooms.com) and is a registered British Association for Counselling and Psychotherapy member. She is a working single mom and has been a meditator and mindfulness user for over twenty-five years. She is also cochair of the Books Committee of the Writer's Guild of Great Britain.